Opening the Energy Gates
of Your Body

Other Books by Bruce Frantzis

Chi Revolution:
Harness the Healing Power of Your Life Force

The Power of Internal Martial Arts and Chi:
Combat and Energy Secrets of Bagua, Tai Chi and Hsing-I

Relaxing Into Your Being (Tao Meditation, Vol. 1):
Chi, Breathing and Dissolving Inner Pain

The Great Stillness (Tao Meditation, Vol. 2):
Awareness, Moving Meditation and Sex Qigong

Tao of Letting Go:
Meditation for Modern Living

Tai Chi: Health for Life

Dragon and Tiger Medical Qigong:
Develop Health and Energy in 7 Simple Movements

Bagua and Tai Chi:
Exploring the Potential of Chi, Martial Arts, Meditation and the I-Ching

Opening the Energy Gates of Your Body

Qigong for Lifelong Health

Bruce Frantzis

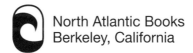

North Atlantic Books
Berkeley, California

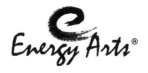

Published by
Energy Arts, Inc.
P.O. Box 99 Fairfax, CA 94978-0099

Distributed by
North Atlantic Books
P.O. Box 12327 Berkeley, CA 94712

North Atlantic Books is part of the Society for the Study of Native Arts and Sciences, a nonprofit educational corporation whose goals are to develop an educational and cross-cultural perspective linking various
scientific, social and artistic fields; to nurture a holistic view of arts, sciences, humanities and healing; and to
publish and distribute literature on the relationship of mind, body and nature.

The following trademarks are used under license by Energy Arts, Inc. from Bruce Frantzis:
Frantzis Energy Arts® system; Mastery Without Mystery®; Longevity Breathing® program;
Opening the Energy Gates of Your Body™ Qigong; Marriage of Heaven and Earth™ Qigong;
Bend the Bow™ Spinal Qigong; Spiraling Energy Body™ Qigong; Gods Playing in the Clouds™ Qigong;
Living Taoism™ Collection; Chi Rev Workout™; Heartchi® and *Energy Arts*

Cover design: Meagan Miller
Cover photos: Coyote Butte's Sandstone Stripes © Joseph Shon: ChormoSohm Inc./CORBIS
Silhouette photo by Don Kellogg, model Dorothy Fitzer. Back cover photo: Richard Marks

Printed and bound in the United States of America

PLEASE NOTE: The practice of martial arts and the meditative arts may carry risks. The instructions and advice
printed in this book are in not any way intended as a substitute for medical, mental or emotional counseling
with a licensed physician or healthcare provider. The reader should consult a professional before undertaking
this or any other martial arts, movement, meditative arts, health or exercise program to reduce the chance of
injury or any other harm that may result from pursuing the instructions and advice presented in this book. Any
physical or other distress experienced during or after any exercise should not be ignored, and should be
brought to the attention of a healthcare professional. The creators and publishers of this book disclaim any
liabilities for loss in connection with following any of the practices, exercises and advice contained in this
book, and their implementation are at the discretion, decision and risk of the reader.

ISBN 13: 978-1-58394-146-1
Library of Congress Cataloging-in-Publication Data
Frantzis, Bruce Kumar.
  Opening the energy gates of your body: qigong for lifelong health/
Bruce Kumar Frantzis.– 2nd ed.
     p. cm.
  Includes bibliographical references and index.
  Summary: "Bruce Frantzis demystifies the fundamental principles of qigong and provides a comprehensive
exercise program with detailed illustrations to increase life energy, improve health, boost sports performance,
and combat stress and aging."–Provided by Publisher.
  ISBN 1-58394-146-0 (trade paper)
1. Qi gong. I. Title.
   RA781.8.F73 2006
   613.7'148–dc22

                                                                          2005032082

              4 5 6 7 8 9 10 11 / 14 13

This book is dedicated to the wonder of the Tao, which lets all things come into being.

My profound thanks to all my teachers in the Orient, without whom it would have been impossible for me to learn and share the information presented here.

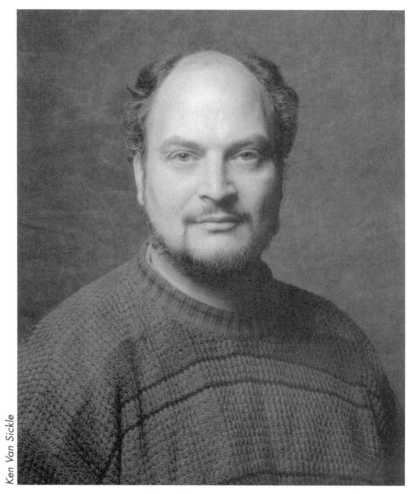

Ken Van Sickle

The author, Bruce Frantzis

Contents

Acknowledgments

My gratitude goes to many. First, to Liu Hung Chieh, a man whose intense impact on me cannot be described with words. Without Liu, I could never have learned or understood qigong so completely. To all of my students, whose genuine interest was the motivation for writing this book. To Natalie Albert and Jan Lang, who first talked me into teaching them this material in the West in New York City in 1972.

Many people helped in the actual creation of the first edition of this book: David Barbero, Craig Barnes, Mary Christianson, Alan Dougall, Jonathan Finegold, Eric Hoffman, Helena Kierulf, Beverly Kune, Brian Lee, Donna Lubell, Susan Rabinowitz, Christine Richardson, Don Rubbo, Bill Ryan, Jim Stegenga, Ken Van Sickle and Michael Vasquez. Special thanks to editor Stuart Kenter, without whom this book would never have been finished.

Thanks to illustrators Kurt Schulten and Michael McKee and the following photographers: Don Kellogg, Mette Heinz, Richard Marks, Ken Van Sickle, Bill Walters, Larry Horton, Sara Barchus, Craig Barnes, Caroline Frantzis, Hideki Matsuoka and Anthony Ortega.

Thanks to the following for their help with the revised second edition: Bill Ryan, founder of Brookline Tai Chi and Toward Harmony Tai Chi and Qigong, for his suggestions for changes in new chapters; Judy Pruzinsky for typing the manuscript into the computer; Linda Olstein for her copy edits of early versions of the revised manuscript; Diane Rapaport for editorial and production management; editor George Glassman; Susan Tillman, editorial assistance; Lisa Petty, GirlVibe, Inc., for design and production; indexer Ken DellaPenta; Meagan Miller for creating the book's cover; Damian Gordon for graphics assistance; photo models Elisha Colas, Brian Cookman, Dorothy Fitzer, Cleophas Gaillard, Aischa Huebner, Leslie Lowe, Kaua Pereira, Ellen Pucciarelli and Alistair Shanks; and to my publisher, Richard Grossinger of North Atlantic Books, for encouraging me to write the revised edition. Thanks also to North Atlantic staff members Anastasia McGhee, Paula Morrison and Mark Oimet, for their help and advice.

Finally, thanks to my wife, Caroline, for her editorial and book production assistance and for her never-ending inspiration and support.

Note to the Reader

The practical side of Taoism is little known in the West. Most of the books about Taoism that are available in English are broad philosophical or poetic treatises (such as those by Lao Tse and Chuang Tse) that do not reveal the actual Taoist methods by which people can manifest Taoist ideals in their daily lives. The end purpose of all Taoist methods resides in Taoist meditation and alchemy, where an individual ultimately understands and becomes one with the mystery of the universe. Along the way, Taoists cherish practices that raise the human being from the "Inferior Man" to the "Superior Man" of the I Ching, who is the only one capable of realizing the Tao.[1]

There are many ways to refine one's body, emotions, and mental and psychic energy en route to becoming—from the Taoist point of view—a mature, balanced adult. I have followed the methodology of the warrior/healer/priest, learning along that road martial arts, qigong, Chinese medicine, Taoist sexual practices and Taoist meditation and philosophy. Taoist friends of mine have taken various paths—qigong, painting, calligraphy, geomancy, and mental pursuits, including the primary method of meditation to move towards the Tao. What all Taoist practitioners of whatever tradition have in common, however, is qigong.

To rise from "inferior" to "superior" in the Taoist manner, the energy of one's body and emotions needs to be strong and balanced. If you are ill, qigong will provide you with a means to become healthy; if your mind is disordered, qigong can give you a way to attain balanced discipline and perseverance. If you are healthy, qigong can raise your energy level, release suppressed talents, and prepare the body/mind/spirit to succeed in Taoist meditation. All people are born "inferior"—it is only through great effort and genuine humility that a person transcends. All sane people wish to be healthy and strong; all those interested in spirituality wish to attain their true nature. In Taoism, qigong is the first basic method for achieving these very human goals.

The techniques of Opening the Energy Gates of Your Body Qigong form the foundation for the health and power aspects of both the Taoist warrior and the qigong healer traditions. By learning and practicing the material in this book, you will be taking the most important first step to genuine lifelong health and vibrancy.

If this world of ours can gain a little more internal balance from books such as this one, that is enough.

---

[1] The Chinese term "Man" should be taken to mean both men and women—humankind.

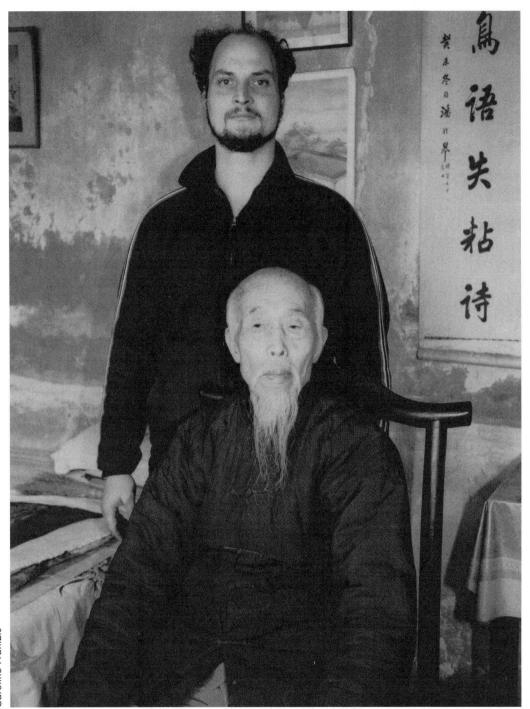

鳥語失粘詩

Caroline Frantzis

Bruce Frantzis was a disciple of the late Taoist Lineage Master Liu Hung Chieh, without whom this book could never have been written. The author wishes to express his deep gratitude to Liu for passing down the ancient traditions of qigong, internal martial arts and Taoist meditation.

Foreword by Stuart Kenter

Bruce Frantzis: The Path of Warrior/ Healer/Priest

Hong Kong: In Search of the Elusive Chi Power

The dream of every serious student of tai chi,[1] qigong[2] and the martial arts is to study with an authentic Oriental grandmaster who will reveal all the secrets of these arts. These secrets of internal power are not taught to the general public, but are privately transmitted only to select family members or inner-circle disciples. In China, being accepted as the disciple of a grandmaster is the equivalent in the West of being admitted to do postdoctoral work at Harvard or Oxford with the most brilliant professor in one's field.

Bruce Kumar Frantzis is one of the very few Westerners who genuinely has been able to achieve this dream. In an odyssey through various martial arts that began in 1961, his ambition was always to study with a lineage grandmaster. Like other Westerners who sought this path, Frantzis was constantly thwarted throughout those years by the tightly closed door of Mainland China, a country where he was both isolated and subject to the harsh consequences of traumatic political upheavals. His frustration was intensified by an unrelenting Oriental prejudice: the unspoken agreement that the most secret teachings should not be given to Westerners.

It was not until the summer of 1981 that one of Frantzis' teachers in Hong Kong

---

[1] Tai Chi (pronounced tie jee) is an ancient Chinese system of movements based upon the development of the chi (life force) within the body. Cultivated chi can be used to rejuvenate the body, heal illness and injuries, maintain health, and enhance spiritual capacities. Tai chi may also be used as a highly effective system of self-defense.

[2] Qigong (pronounced chee gung) is the art and practice of internal energy development.

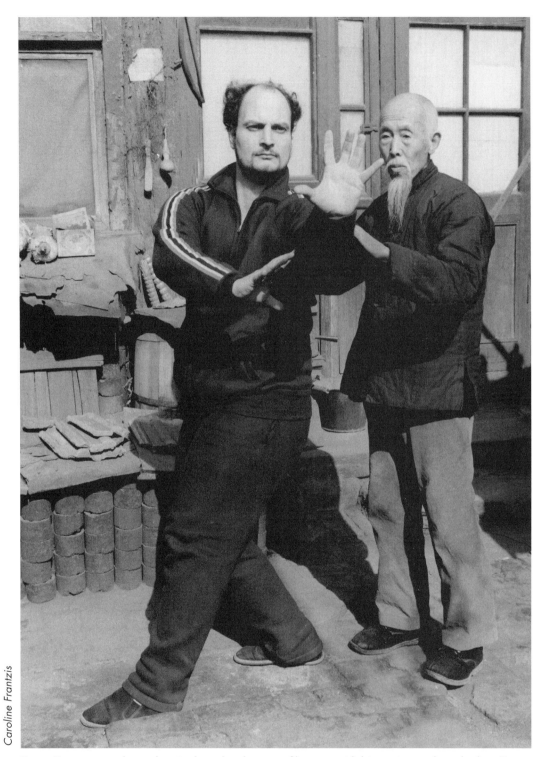

Caroline Frantzis

Bruce Frantzis works on the single palm change of bagua with his main teacher, the late Taoist Lineage Master Liu Hung Chieh, in Beijing, China.

consented to give him a letter of introduction to his own master in Beijing, a man named Liu Hung Chieh (pronounced Lee-oh Hung Jee-eh). This letter contained potential that excited Frantzis greatly. He had already been invited there by the Beijing Institute of Physical Education to study tai chi chuan (*Chuan:* fist).

During that summer in Beijing, Frantzis spent his mornings studying the national simplified system of tai chi, push hands and weapons. The instruction emphasized the health aspects of tai chi over its martial arts applications, and it is here that Frantzis gained a deep knowledge and respect for tai chi as a comprehensive healthcare system. At the conclusion of this course, Frantzis was the first Westerner to be certified in Beijing by the Chinese government to teach the complete system of tai chi chuan. Frantzis went on to develop tai chi and qigong into a viable healthcare program useful to the West.

In the afternoons, Frantzis would study with Grandmaster Liu in his home. After the tai chi course was completed, Frantzis would study in the mornings and afternoons with Liu, a standard practice that would continue throughout the time that Frantzis was living in Beijing.

Beijing: Grandmaster Liu Hung Chieh

Frantzis studied for a total of three years with Grandmaster Liu Hung Chieh, who was in his eighties. Liu had an intriguing past.

He had lived and studied with the founder of Wu style tai chi, Wu Jien Chuan, and he had been the youngest member of the original Beijing Bagua Zhang[3] School. When he was only in his thirties, Liu was declared enlightened by the Tien Tai School of Buddhism, after which he spent ten years studying with Taoists in the mountains of Western China. He was a lineage holder in tai chi, hsing-i[4] and bagua as well as an adept in Taoist qigong and meditation practices.

Like many of the traditional martial artists, Liu was not a public person. Since the revolution in China in 1949, he had taught hsing-i and bagua to just one man—Frantzis' teacher

---

[3] Bagua (pronounced bah-gwa) is the most sophisticated and mysterious of the Chinese internal martial arts. Based upon manifesting the energies of the *I Ching* (*Book of Changes*), it is the only internal martial art that is completely Taoist in conception and practice. It is primarily a spiritual art that is at the same time considered to be an unsurpassed system of self-defense. It is thought by many to be the highest and most effective of all the Chinese internal arts (*Ba:* eight; *Gua:* trigrams; *Zhang:* palm.)

[4] Hsing-i (pronounced shing-ee) is a major attack-oriented Chinese internal martial art based on developing chi for health, rejuvenation and power. It is known for making practitioners physically and mentally strong, enabling them to accomplish their goals. *Hsing* means "form" and *I* means the "intention of the mind." Whenever the mind moves, the body creates a form and the goal is achieved.

in Hong Kong, Bai Hua. When Frantzis had asked Bai Hua if Liu would take him on as a student in Beijing, the instructor replied, "Who knows? He teaches virtually no one and it's impossible to predict what he will do."

Liu was cordial to Frantzis at their first meeting. Frantzis realized immediately that the twenty years he had spent immersed in the martial arts and meditation would only serve as a foundation to studying with this man. Well over twice Frantzis' age and less than half his size, Liu was able to pick Frantzis up and move him any way he wished. Frantzis, on the other hand, was literally unable to move even Liu's little finger. Frantzis, who was considered to be a "young master" in Hong Kong and Taiwan, was duly impressed. Liu told him, "There is more to having energy than just being big."

During the years that Frantzis studied with Liu, he was frequently able to observe the results of the Taoist rejuvenation techniques that the older man practiced. These would seem to change Liu from an old man to a young one in the space of a few hours or days. The transformation was amazing, and Frantzis saw this control over the aging process as the mark of a true master.

Frantzis requested Liu to teach him bagua. Instruction entailed the most strenuous energy work that Frantzis had yet undertaken. After the lessons, he would be so fatigued that Liu let him lie on his own bed, entertaining him with stories of Buddhism and Taoism, and teaching him meditation. Years later, Liu revealed that the only reason he had consented to teach Frantzis was that his arrival had been presaged in a dream. Liu had had five prophetic dreams in his life, all of which had come to pass. Like many of the older Taoists, Liu believed in karmic connections being fulfilled, and he felt deeply that such a connection existed between himself and Frantzis. It was Liu who began to teach Frantzis the deeper internal secrets of qigong and other Taoist energy arts found in this and other books Frantzis has written.[5]

New York City: The First Training Ground

Born at the end of the 1940s in New York City, Frantzis was a fat, clumsy kid who at the age of twelve witnessed a fellow student get badly injured in a fight at school. This event had a powerful effect on him, and an ad in a subway that promised "Fear No Man!" led him to his first judo class. Shortly thereafter, he also began to practice karate, jiu-jitsu, aikido, and Zen Buddhism.

---

[5] See Appendix G.

He was fourteen when he became involved with Zen. At that time, he used it primarily as a tool to eliminate hesitation from his karate and weapons forms. His interest in meditation at this young age was primarily focused on training the mind for martial arts rather than for spiritual growth. Even without the spiritual component, however, Frantzis claims that Zen provided him with a one-pointedness that led to the strength to move through obstacles.

His early years were concentrated on learning the Japanese martial arts. He had earned black belts in jiu-jitsu, karate, and aikido even before his first trip to the Orient, and another in judo soon thereafter. Following the recommendation of his jiu-jitsu teacher, he also studied shiatsu (Japanese acupressure massage), and he practiced this type of bodywork throughout high school. Both aikido and shiatsu utilize *ki* (the Japanese word for chi), or life energy; aikido for power and shiatsu for healing. Clearly Frantzis' interest in, and emphasis on, the subject of health started at a very early age.

By age eighteen, it had become clear to him that, in order to learn the essence of the Oriental martial, healing and meditation arts, he would have to find their source. This desire led to sixteen years of study abroad: eleven years in China, three in Japan, and two in India.

Still, his teenage years in the martial arts were primarily motivated largely by a fascination with destruction. He was, at the time, preoccupied with how to injure the human body. Paradoxically, even his ongoing interest in health and meditation was, during this period, expressed in terms of violence: Zen meditation became to him a way of destroying the nonsense layers of his mind. Doing massage became a way to vanquish people's aches and pains. It was not until later, in his twenties, that he changed, allowing his interest in health and well-being to dominate completely. At that time, he also became seriously involved with learning how to apply the techniques of the martial, healing, and meditation arts to preserve the useful aspects of body, mind, and spirit, keeping them from harm.

This transition began in China. Here, Frantzis witnessed firsthand elderly practitioners of qigong who were healthier and more vital than people half their age. He was awed, at first, by the physical techniques of qigong. Then, when he began to learn the actual qigong methods of working directly with energy, he understood: here was a way of *preserving* and *increasing* strength and vitality. He noticed that all those he saw practicing—himself included—grew stronger with age, and more content. In the Chinese hospital clinics where for many years he practiced qigong therapeutic massage (*qigong tui na*, pronounced chee gung tway na), he watched people who had been weak and sickly all their lives become—through qigong—men and women of obviously superior health and strength. He saw many who were neurotic, mentally disturbed or prone to extremes of anger, depression, anxiety or fear become calm, stable, and balanced through qigong. He witnessed qigong elevate dull minds to intelligence and perceptivity. To Frantzis, the Chinese arts worked demonstrably better, and made more sense, than much of what Western medicine or athletic workouts had to offer.

Tokyo: The Path through Aikido

In 1967, at the age of eighteen, Frantzis traveled to Japan, where he enrolled at Sophia University in Tokyo. His primary interest was still in the hard styles of the martial arts, such as karate. He had the good fortune—from 1967 to 1969—to study with the founder of aikido, Morihei Ueshiba. He was an extraordinary man, one who had unmistakably reached an advanced level of chi development. During the last few months of his life, too weak to walk, he had to be carried into the dojo (practice hall). Yet, even in this condition, he was able to stand up and suddenly muster the energy to throw his strongest students as if they were rag dolls. After practice, he would again be carried back to his bed. Frantzis took such episodes as a graphic example of how the life force transcended mere flesh.

While Ueshiba passed on the physical techniques and spiritual philosophy of aikido to his students, Frantzis felt that none of them had attained Ueshiba's remarkable level of chi. It had been a widely known but little discussed fact within the dojo that after Ueshiba had spent a long time in China as a monk, his entire technique changed: it went from aiki-jitsu to aikido (do is the Japanese word for Tao). That is, it went from a system based on jiu-jitsu to one based on the use of ki, or chi. At this juncture in his career, Frantzis had black belts in five of the Japanese martial arts. He had visited many of the top Japanese teachers. None of them, in his view, had Ueshiba's tremendous chi power. Frantzis wanted to find out what chi practices Ueshiba had learned in China.

Taiwan: The Astonishing Wang Shu Jin

Yet another experience pointed in the direction of China when Frantzis visited Taiwan in 1968. There he met Wang Shu Jin,[6] an internal martial arts master who had come to Taiwan from the city of Tianjin in Mainland China. Wang was in his seventies and—at five

---

[6] Wang's name is written as Wang Shu-Chin in many English language publications.

feet eight inches tall—overweight at 250-plus pounds. Nonetheless, he proved to be physically faster than the much younger Frantzis, whom he could throw or knock across the room at will.

In their conversation, Wang maintained that karate had inferior fighting technique and insisted that actual prolonged karate practice itself would make your body old and damaged before its time. Frantzis, who had studied karate for most of his life, disagreed vehemently, which resulted—as such differences of opinion between martial artists often do—in a challenge. Wang invited Frantzis to test the reality of his view.

What Frantzis remembers best about that fight was that he only ended up hurting his hands and feet on various parts of Wang's body, and that Wang had the disconcerting habit of ending up behind him several times during the fight, tapping him on the shoulder. Etched deeply in Frantzis' mind is the moment in their match when Wang walked slowly toward him, eyes half shut. At that moment, Frantzis relates that he actually began to fear for his life. He backed up against a wall, braced himself, and heel-kicked Wang as forcefully as he could in the solar plexus. The kick simply woke Wang up and made him mad. He tapped Frantzis on the head. Frantzis felt a bolt of electricity jolt through his body and the next thing he knew, he was suddenly, and to his complete surprise, on the floor.

Frantzis began to practice with Wang's 5 a.m. class in Tai Chung Park. About a week into the sessions, an old man who was a fellow student, asked Frantzis if he wanted to "play." This elderly man was short and thin, a student after all, and Frantzis felt a bit uneasy, not wanting to take advantage of him. He acquiesced, however, and after being hit a few times, decided his concern was misplaced. He went after the old man as hard as he knew how. The fellow had no trouble handling Frantzis as an opponent. Frantzis was stunned at this turn of events. While he was standing there dazed, the man's wife came over and asked if she could have a go. After a year in Japan, Frantzis did not know how to refuse such offers. He found to his amazement that she could spar with him on the level of any top competitive Japanese second-degree black belt in karate.

Frantzis became so utterly depressed over this experience with the elderly couple that he seriously considered quitting the martial arts completely. That Master Wang Shu-jin could beat him was one thing; that these seemingly average and elderly students could beat him was something else. By this time, he had been a black belt for four years by this time. He had been training in Japan for eight hours a day. Yet he felt he had missed the boat. Were they going to bring out five-year-olds to beat him next? Should he have started when he was three instead of twelve? Should he have been practicing *fourteen* hours a day?

He had the opportunity, a few days later, to converse with this elderly couple from Taiwan. (By then Frantzis was fluent in Japanese, which many elderly Taiwanese also spoke). They had come to study with Wang seven years previously because the husband suffered greatly from arthritis. He was initially concerned with regaining his health, not with learning martial arts. After three years of practicing tai chi, bagua, hsing-i, and qigong, however, he was loose and his back had straightened so felt he could cease practicing. Six months after he stopped, his symptoms recurred. When he resumed practice, the symptoms went into remission.

The day before this conversation, trying to regain some of his lost confidence, Frantzis had fought—and was duly beaten by—some of Wang's teenage students. It became more than obvious to him that *all* of Wang's students had reached a superlative level of both health and power through the development of their chi. Frantzis' thought changed direction: if each and every one of Wang's students could attain these ends, then he could too. His commitment to study the Chinese internal arts with Wang was cemented then and there.

Wang began to explain the difference between the internal and external martial arts. Whereas the external arts develop the bones, muscles, and outer physique, the internal arts concentrate on the development of chi. Qigong and the internal arts of tai chi, hsing-i and bagua enable one to work with the energies of the body, so that chi becomes as tangible as a solid object. The energy field in the air becomes as real to a qigong or internal arts practitioner as the water in the ocean is to a swimmer.

Before the internal arts were ever used for self-defense, they were part of Taoist yoga, where their chief purpose was to heal the body, calm the mind,

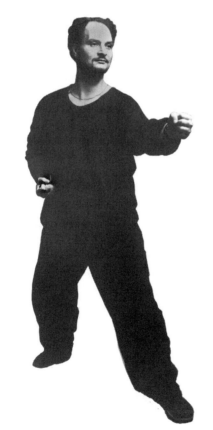

Ken Van Sickle

Bruce Frantzis demonstrates a hsing-i punch.

promote longevity, and form the physical foundation for higher meditation practices. The internal arts are based on beautiful flowing movements that develop structural integrity, sound body mechanics, and a strong sense of physical and psychic power. The nineteen-year-old Frantzis would never forget the words directed to him by the seventy-year-old Wang: "I can eat more than you can, I have more sexual vitality than you do, I can move and fight better than you can, I never get sick, and you call yourself healthy? There is more to being healthy than merely being young. Chi can teach you all of this." Frantzis recognized the truth in Wang's words and studied with him on and off for ten years.

Frantzis returned to Sophia University in Tokyo. From 1968 to 1971, while still taking courses there, he pursued his study of internal arts with the hsing-i master, Kenichi Sawai, and with various students that Wang Shu Jin had in Japan. He was also fortunate enough during this period to have encountered an old Chinese doctor who taught him qigong tui na, a Chinese bodywork system whose fundamentals he was able to master over a period of two years. Frantzis would later learn much more about this system and use it in his clinical work. With this doctor, Frantzis was introduced for the first time to a man who could consistently transmit the chi energy from his own hands to cure illnesses and repair the bodies of others. During his third year in Japan, Frantzis became a special karate research student in Okinawa, where he concentrated further on karate and weapons systems. Here, at the veritable birthplace of karate, he keenly felt the absence of practices that developed chi and improved health, as well as a lack of many of the most sophisticated martial arts techniques. He came to a realization that caused him to give up the study of purely external hard styles for good. From this point on, he focused all his efforts solely on the internal martial arts and qigong.

India: Meditation as Chi Cultivation

From the Taoism that he learned from Wang Shu Jin in Taiwan, Frantzis knew that energy cultivation could be one of the basic methods of meditation. Since legend dictated that Bodhidharma had brought the martial arts and meditation from India to the Shaolin Temple in China in the fifth century A.D., Frantzis, always an avid seeker of original sources, decided to go straight to the Indian source. (He had been unaware at that time of the historical fact that China possessed both martial arts and a highly honed chi development methodology centuries before Bodhidharma's visit.)

In 1971, after four-and-a-half years in the Orient, he came back to the United States. Deeply disappointed by the Oriental teachers he encountered in America (as Frantzis saw it, they either withheld information, did not have genuine knowledge to impart in the first place or were unable to convey what they did have because of language difficulties), he decided to return once more to Asia, the "Harvard" of energy development. Until 1987, when he anchored himself permanently in the United States, Frantzis spent years alternating between Asia and the West. He earned his living by teaching qigong and the internal martial arts in the United States and Europe, as well as practicing the healing art of qigong tui na. In 1972, after a six-month stint of teaching tai chi in America, he departed for India.

He went first to an ashram in southern India to learn the techniques of pranayama yoga,[7] which works directly with life energy. He practiced in the classical manner—using breath, mantras,[8] and mudras[9]—four sessions a day, three hours a session. After three months of this intensity, Frantzis says that he was able to "awaken the Kundalini shakti." This is a spiritual force that begins the process of purifying the consciousness, eventually resulting in enlightenment. In northern India, Frantzis studied Tantric Kundalini meditation with Guru Shiv Om-Tirth of Rishikesh, an experience that enabled him to comprehend the fundamental energetic similarities and differences between the Chinese and Indian systems of energy development.

Frantzis knew that both the Indian and Chinese practices, if implemented correctly, could heal and increase longevity through development and control of the life force. Both systems had been proven by the test of time and both had undergone literally thousands of years of testing and refinement. The main difference that Frantzis perceived between the two systems at the level of health resided in the nature of their practice: the Chinese system is concerned with body motion, the unceasing flow of energy, like water in a stream, whereas the Indian methods use postures with distinct beginnings and ends, and pauses between each posture. The difference is more profound, on an experiential level, than it might seem. Tai chi and qigong are active; yoga is passive. Yoga seems to give greater flexibility, whereas tai chi builds greater power and integration of movement. Yet both are similar in that genuine hatha yoga teaches pranayama with the postures—the postures open the body and the pranayama works with the energy. Genuine Chinese internal arts, in comparison, utilize certain movements—motions that encourage internal energy circulation.

---

[7] *Prana*: breath; *yama*: to control or develop. Pranayama is the Indian parallel to qigong. Beginning with breath control techniqes, one eventually learns in this practice to control the movement of internal life force energy.

[8] Chants using specialized sounds cause specific energies to be released at the physical, mental and spiritual levels.

[9] Hand and finger positions that evoke energies and mental states in the practitioner.

However without internal energy work, the amount of energy gained in either system is relatively small. Frantzis believes that, in the vast majority of instances, the teaching of yoga, tai chi and qigong in the West fails to include the internal components. Sole emphasis on the external martial arts, or the external movements of tai chi, or the external postures of yoga, Frantzis maintains, can only develop a severely limited amount of chi.

The two systems are by no means mutually exclusive. Frantzis believes that they can be practiced simultaneously to beneficial effect. For those who are currently practicing yoga, the Chinese arts can prove a wonderful adjunct, accelerating the process of clearing obstructions and developing energy. Although while studying in India, he was able to achieve many of the most difficult postures of hatha yoga, Frantzis never found this practice as satisfying as the movement arts.

There was one aspect of his India experience that Frantzis felt uneasy about: the concept of the guru. Worship of the guru plays a pivotal role in the Indian traditions, the guru being God's direct representative on earth. As divine agents, gurus are treated with a deference and reverence that very few Westerners would accord to a living person. Though the Chinese tradition also accords a greater respect to teachers than one finds in the West, Taoist masters (bear in mind that not all Chinese masters are Taoist) are considered to be custodians of ancient wisdom. The relationship between student and teacher in the Taoist way is more like a respected friend helping a friend than a godlike master helping out a mere mortal. The Taoists consider everybody to be one in the Tao and they speak of being friends in the Tao. Consequently, Frantzis' training under the Taoists had a much lighter feeling for him than his training under gurus.

In India, Frantzis was able to formulate a comparative perspective on the world's two classic systems of internal energy. He assimilated a great deal of valuable knowledge on meditation and chi there. Unfortunately, he also was infected with a nearly fatal case of hepatitis.

Taiwan, Hong Kong, Poona, Beijing: From Consummate Fighter to Consummate Healer

The extremely virulent form of hepatitis Frantzis contracted in India killed two close friends and left his own liver severely damaged. He is convinced that without the energy work learned from tai chi and qigong, he too would have died in India. His situation was grim. He lay on a hospital bed barely able to move. The Indian doctor who examined Frantzis told him that he was in danger of dying. He recognized the truth of what the physician said and knew that he would in fact die unless he did something. He crawled out of his bed and, shaking all the while, stood and forced himself to do tai chi and qigong movements. The pain throughout his body was fierce, but he persevered until he finally collapsed back onto the bed. He slept continuously for three days. When he awoke, he knew that he would live.

When he was able to travel, he returned to Taiwan. Here he practiced the internal arts with a passion, working with bagua fighting master Hung I Hsiang for a cumulative period of four years. Frantzis is certain that this practice slowly regenerated his liver, allowing him to continue his martial studies. He explored the half-internal, half-external Kung Fu styles of Eight Drunken Immortals, Northern Praying Mantis, Fukien White Crane, Northern Monkey, and Wing Chun. He realized that many of the truly superior martial arts teachers from mainland China were very old, and felt that this might be his last chance to learn many of these arts well, before they faded completely from the face of the earth. During this incred-

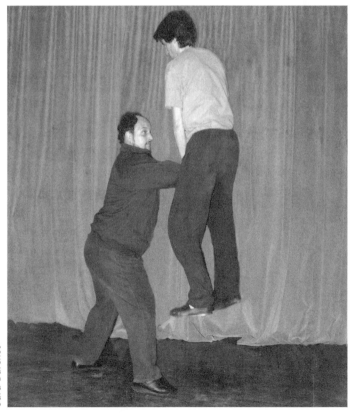

Sara Barchus

Bruce Frantzis discharges energy in order to uproot his opponent. This advanced technique is commonly found in tai chi push hands and other internal martial arts.

ibly intense period of concentration on the fighting arts, Frantzis squeezed out time to study medical qigong for treating specific diseases. He paid special attention to qigong for nerve and spine regeneration. With his energy level continually increasing from his practices, he was also able to devote time to studying meditation with Taoists, whose emphasis was on clearing negative emotions from the body and the mind.

Toward the end of 1975, Frantzis flew back to Manhattan, teaching semi-privately and treating many of his patients with qigong exercises and qigong tui na. He was still unwilling to teach large groups publicly, both out of respect for the Oriental tradition and because he felt that he did not know enough to teach in this way and would not be able to monitor the progress of his students since he was traveling back and forth from Asia.

In the United States this time around, he became acutely aware of the significance of stress in American life, and of the vast numbers who were burning themselves out through overwork and worry. He thought a great deal about how to apply his Taoist training to this problem but knew that there were gaps in his medical education. Many of the internal organ structural health problems he encountered were beyond his abilities to deal with as a qigong healer. He kept a careful log of all the weak areas in his training and when he returned to the Orient within a year, he attempted to find the missing medical links he required.

His search for insight into the emotions and their impact on stress-related conditions took him to Poona, India, in 1977. There, he continued his Tantric studies while simultaneously working with a group that explored the connection between emotions, the psychological realms, meditation and chi, integrating Kundalini methods with New Age psychotherapeutic techniques. This research provided Frantzis with excellent information on how the workings of the Western mind fit into the Oriental energy framework.

By late 1977, he was back in Taiwan, devoting twelve hours a day to the internal arts, refining his bagua, immersing himself in Taoist and Tantric meditation, and developing a sharp interest in processing bound emotional energy. He continued his work on studying the spine and nervous system. Although he completed an advanced acupuncture degree in Hong Kong in 1978, he chose instead to concentrate on qigong therapy rather than practice acupuncture.

In late 1979, he moved to Denver, Colorado, opening a private school that was restricted to a few continuing students. It was not until after studying with Grandmaster Liu in Beijing that Frantzis was confident enough of his mastery of the internal components of qigong to teach public workshops and write books on the subject. After enjoying considerable success in the full-contact fighting arena for years, Frantzis now began to shift away from fighting to focus in depth on healing and meditation. By the end of the 1970s and through his subsequent years in Beijing, Frantzis had continued to refine his fighting techniques, however his primary emphasis had markedly and irrevocably changed. Indeed, during the summer of 1981, the seminal time when he worked diligently with Grandmaster Liu Hung Chieh in Beijing, he was so deeply immersed in his training he never even visited the Forbidden City, even though it was a five minute walk from Liu's house.

In fall of 1981, Bruce Frantzis returned to Denver, where he quietly resumed teaching and training instructors, and was nearly crippled for life.

Denver: The Crisis of Self-Healing

In early 1982, Frantzis was involved in a bad automobile accident. He suffered massive injury to his spine. Two vertebrae were badly cracked, a few more had hairline fractures, many of the spinal ligaments and tendons were torn, and all his vertebrae were knocked out of alignment. Surgeons pressured him to have a spinal fusion, which Frantzis, through his pain, impolitely refused. His years of exposure to qigong and qigong tui na had taught him that, given his condition, once his spine was cut open, the chi of his body would never be as full again. Keeping the surgeons at bay, Frantzis began doing qigong flat on his back eight to ten hours a day.

Miracles did not occur. It was a long, hard ordeal regenerating his spine with these techniques. Complications arose. Frantzis speaks of how the shattering of his spine neutralized every psychological control mechanism he had. All the darkest forces suppressed in the depths of his mind surfaced. Without his years of centering work in meditation, Frantzis was sure that he would have gone over the edge, sentenced to life in a mental hospital. Instead, he held on.

However the emotional experience on top of the constant nerve pain made life unbearable, both for himself and for those around him. His sudden loss of physical strength and ability, the broken pride as an athlete, was a devastating blow. He fell into a profound depression, losing all interest in tai chi and unable to do bagua because of the pain. He knew he had to do something about his mental outlook. The feeling of being useless to himself and his students could not continue. When qigong practice finally repaired his spine enough to be able to move to some extent, Frantzis participated in various mind/body therapies in Colorado and Oregon. They helped somewhat, reinforcing his mental stability. However, no matter how effective a psychological therapy may be, round-the-clock nerve pain created emotional havoc. The psychological work was not enough.

Frantzis tried all the physical therapies, including chiropractic, deep tissue work, Rolfing, acupuncture, massage, and a variety of movement therapies. They, too, helped marginally, abating the pain for a day or two, but it always returned. When it became clear that the alternatives available to him in the West would not permanently restore him, Frantzis did what he had always done—he went to China to search, this time for the appropriate healing technology to make his own body whole.

Beijing Again: The Final Lesson with Liu

When Frantzis arrived in Beijing in the Summer of 1983, Liu was in meditation retreat and unavailable to work with him. Fortunately, because of another letter from his teacher in Hong Kong, Bai Hua, Frantzis was able instead to study the inner technology of Yang style tai chi with Lin Du Ying[10] in Xiamen, Fujien Province. Although Frantzis had studied the Yang style of tai chi with many teachers, including Yang Shao Jung (the great-grandson of Yang Lu Chan, the original Yang, who founded the Yang style of tai chi), he had great respect for Lin Du Ying, deeming him the most exceptional practitioner of the Yang style he had ever seen. Since Frantzis had been accepted as a formal disciple, he was given the information openly. He felt that it was an honor to be allowed to receive this tai chi transmission from Lin.

When after nine months Liu was finally available, Frantzis joined him. While his practice of the Yang form had eased the pain in his neck and upper back, the rest of his body still hurt. Liu prescribed Wu style tai chi. This style emphasizes soft healing and meditation; it strengthens the body and clears the mind. Within months, practicing the Wu form obliterated the pain in Frantzis' middle and lower back.

Liu then began teaching Frantzis Taoist meditation, twice a day, in two to three hour sessions. Once Frantzis' lower back had healed sufficiently, Liu commenced the teaching of bagua and hsing-i, as well as certain qigong methodologies. This training went on for three years, seven days a week, nonstop.

Liu filled in many gaps in Frantzis' esoteric education (accumulated over twenty years) and escorted him to places in the mind he never knew existed. He led Frantzis through all

[10] Lin Du Ying was a disciple of Wu Hui Chuan and Tien Jau Ling, both of whom were top students of Yang Pan Hou, son of Yang Lu Chan, the originator of the Yang style of tai chi. Lin Du Ying taught the Yang style in a very pure manner, in much the same way it was taught a hundred years ago, before it became diluted.

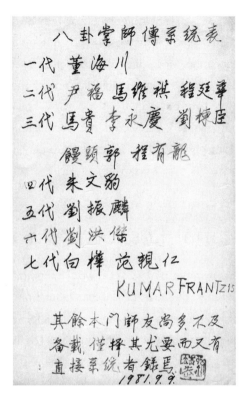

八卦掌師傳系統表
一代 董海川
二代 尹福 馬維祺 程廷華
三代 馬貴 李永慶 劉棟庄
　　　饅頭郭 程有龍
四代 朱文豹
五代 劉振麟
六代 劉洪傑
七代 白樺 范覥仁
　　　KUMAR FRANTZIS

其餘本門師友尚多不及
備載 僅擇其尤要而又有
直接系統者錄焉
1981.9.9.

This certificate from the late Taoist Lineage Master Liu Hung Chieh shows Bruce Kumar Frantzis' place in the seventh generation of bagua lineage masters.

the levels of Taoist meditation practice, into directly experiencing the place where all is unified with the Tao. It was Liu's wish that Frantzis teach not only martial arts and qigong (which, by this time, he was thoroughly qualified to do), but Taoist meditation as well, when Frantzis felt comfortable to do so. It was through Liu that Frantzis was able to organize the qigong system presented in this and other volumes. Liu took the unprecedented step of authorizing a Westerner to impart knowledge locked up in China since antiquity.

On December 1, 1986, Liu died just one day after he finished teaching Frantzis the last palm change of bagua zhang and the final level of Wu style tai chi. He had passed the lineage on to Frantzis. The sadness was overwhelming. Frantzis felt deeply privileged to have met such a man. To have studied with Liu was to have been the recipient of a great and rare gift. After being extended the honor of stirring Liu's ashes, usually an act confined to the immediate family,[11] Frantzis returned home to the United States.

Frantzis' goal in the West was and still is to convey as much as possible of the life-enhancing material he has learned. Liu's generosity gave Frantzis knowledge and confidence, and it is Frantzis' hope that he can bridge cultures by making this knowledge available to people in the West. "The time for secrets," Frantzis says, "is past."

---

[11] Liu had officially adopted Frantzis as his son in a Confucian ceremony.

Introduction to the Revised Edition

In 1987, fresh from learning Taoist energy arts for over a decade in China, I began to write this book's original edition. My goal was to write an easy-to-follow qigong primer that explained what qigong was and provide a set of gentle and enjoyable exercises that people could learn on their own. This volume contains a complete Taoist qigong system—one that has worked for thousands of years. It is the first of the books in my Living Taoism™ collection.

The Growing Acceptance of Qigong in the West

Since its publication in 1993, this book has inspired thousands to take up qigong. This ancient Chinese energy practice combats aging, relaxes the body and mind and improves health.

Now, new circumstances and a growing acceptance of qigong and tai chi have prepared the general public to better accept the increasing relevance of qigong in daily life. When I first wrote the book, I warned of a coming breakdown in our medical care system. Today, that health crisis has arrived. Virtually everyone in the West feels its effects.

I am heartened that doctors and other health practitioners are increasingly recommending these practices to their patients as both preventative systems and methodologies that can improve existing medical conditions. My hope is that the value of qigong, tai chi, yoga and other self-help maintenance systems will be supported at the highest policy levels of government. They are among the lowest cost, most effective and proven ways of benefiting health. These practices are some of the best health insurance policies you can have. They have a long history of successfully reducing chronic illness and stress.

Good health, aging well and relief from stress are goals that each of us can attain.

What the New Edition Contains

Since the first publication of this book, many students have requested that more information be included in a revised edition. Many of those requests mirrored my own desire to add material that would be useful to people who wished to get involved in qigong, as well as for those that wanted to take a long-term look at some of the deeper levels of Opening the Energy Gates of Your Body qigong. Several new chapters have been added to the book and existing chapters have been revised.

New material includes:

- Longevity Breathing techniques.
- Releasing and sinking the chi.
- More details on qigong standing postures.
- Information on sitting postures.
- How to do the Taoist spine stretch while sitting.
- How qigong relates to hatha yoga and other alternative exercise systems, and to such sports as golf and weight training.
- How qigong can lead to spiritual advancement and enhance other religious and meditative practices.
- Advanced aspects of the core exercises.
- Information about , the Taoist system that codifies the full range of energy flow in the body, mind and spirit into 16 components.

In China, qigong and tai chi are mainstream exercises that are practiced by hundreds of millions of people. Many start learning above the age of 50 to improve and maintain their health, reduce stress and combat aging. This is the age when people begin to feel their health slipping and their stress rising. Younger people do not think about their health unless faced with long-term illness or an accident.

In the West, qigong and most other forms of exercise continue to be difficult for those over fifty. The concept of people taking control of their health through regular daily exercise goes against many ingrained habits. This is despite the hard data showing that regular exercise and good diet can help mitigate chronic illness and stress.

Equally, there is growing evidence that qigong and Taoist energy exercises like tai chi can have a potent effect on improving health.

- They have a proven track record that is thousands of years old for being effective health maintenance systems. In the last fifty years, they have helped decrease the stress and improve the health of a mass population in China.

- Western medical studies are proving their efficacy in relieving a whole host of chronic and viral illnesses.
- Practitioners are educating their doctors about the pragmatic benefits they have received. As a result, doctors are learning more about the benefits of qigong and tai chi and are recommending these arts to patients as a viable option.

My hope is that qigong and tai chi become mainstream exercises in the West. People can feel better and experience improvements to their bodies, minds and spirits throughout their lives. There is nothing stagnant about these exercises: learning remains continuous and fresh. What you learn as you continue to practice can be as challenging and demanding as science, sports or any creative discipline and as immensely rewarding.

Don Kellogg

The Third Swing of Opening the Energy Gates of Your Body qigong energizes the heart, lungs, spine and brain.

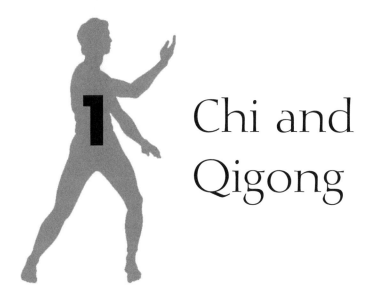

Chi and Qigong

What Is Chi?

Put simply, it is that which gives life. In terms of the body, chi is that which differentiates a corpse from a live human being. To use a Biblical reference, it is that which God breathed into the dust to produce Adam. Chi is the basis of acupuncture; it is the life energy people try desperately to hold onto when they think they are dying.

A strong life force makes a human being totally alive, alert and "present," while a weak force results in sluggishness and fatigue. Energy can be increased in a human being. Consequently, the development of chi can make an ill person robust or a weak person vibrant; it can also enhance mental capacity.

The concept of "life force" is found in most of the ancient cultures of the world. In India, it is called *prana*; in China, *chi*; in Japan, *ki*; for Native Americans, the Great Spirit. For all these cultures, and others as well, the idea of life force is or was central to their forms of medicine and healing.

What Is Qigong?

Qigong, which literally means "energy work," is the practice of learning to control the movement of the life force internally, using only the mind to direct energy in the body. Physical movement may be used, but is not required. As such, it is an internal exercise. The qigong practices presented here include many of the ancient Chinese techniques for increasing life energy. Increased life energy in turn manifests in a variety of ways, from improved physical health to greater mental clarity and spiritual attainment. Regular practice of these exercises will lead to a body/mind that is functionally younger, so that one's "golden years" are truly golden, rather than rusty.

China's 3,000-Year-Old System of Self-Healing

The effectiveness of qigong has been proven in China by its beneficial impact on the health of millions of people over thousands of years. Developing the life force, or chi, is the focus of Taoism, China's original religion/philosophy. The Taoists are the same people who brought acupuncture, Chinese herbal medicine, bone setting, and the yin/yang concept to the world. Unfortunately, most of the specifics of these valuable contributions have until just recently been blocked from Western awareness by immense cultural and language barriers. These barriers are beginning to break down to an extent in acupuncture, but with regard to qigong they are still very much in place. This book on the methodology of qigong is devised to help knock down these walls.

For most people, the first and foremost benefit of qigong lies in the relief or prevention of chronic health problems. The range of maladies that have been helped by qigong in China include cancer, internal organ ailments, poor circulation, nerve pain, back and joint problems and general physical disease.

Qigong Gives Mental Clarity

Many physical problems are at least partially due to, or aggravated by, mental or emotional stress, so the importance of the inner tranquility developed through qigong cannot be overestimated. The practice of qigong helps manage the stress, anger, depression, morbid thoughts, and general confusion that prey on your mind when your chi is not regulated and balanced. Strengthening and balancing the energy of your mind enhances your ability to detect subtle nuances and to perceive the world and its patterns at ever-increasing levels of complexity. People who do not practice some form of energy development many never acquire these abilities.

The Three Spiritual Treasures

Qigong is also useful on the spiritual level. The ultimate aim of all inner Taoist practices is the alchemical transformation of the body, mind, and spirit, leading to union with the Tao. Feeling the energy of your body makes it possible for you to understand the energy of your thoughts and emotions, and this leads to comprehending the energy of the spirit. From here it is possible to fully understand the energy of meditation or emptiness, and through emptiness it is possible to become one with the Tao.

According to Taoism, every human being contains "the three treasures"—*jing* (sperm/ovary energy, or the essence of the physical body), *chi* (energy, including the thoughts and emotions), and *shen* (spirit or spiritual power). *Wu* (emptiness) gives birth to and integrates the three treasures.

The Taoists use the all-pervasive life energy as the basis of spiritual investigation. The ultimate goal, becoming one with the Tao, has been called many things, such as "enlightenment," "meeting with the Father in Heaven," "reaching Nirvana," and "ultimate understanding." Taoists feel that it is best for one to begin with the energy of the body, then progress through emotions and thoughts to spiritual power, before going for the ultimate.

Popular opinion has it that once you have reached a state of emptiness, you stay there, but this idea is false. You merely become increasingly familiar with this state and learn how to spend more and more time there. As long as you live in a physical body, physical needs continue to exert demands, and dwelling completely in emptiness is not possible. Taoism has developed advanced techniques to work with the energy of wu.

Qigong can be practiced by individuals who only want to become physically healthy and do not care about psychological or spiritual matters. For generations, qigong has been used by martial artists, many of whom remained unconcerned with spiritual development. Nonetheless, all Taoist spiritual practice begins with qigong practice, no matter what level of attainment one wishes to finally achieve.

Clearing Energy Blocks

Many people involved with spiritual disciplines focus their attention on enlightenment, and in the process injure their bodies and agitate their minds. They attempt to train in the higher spiritual disciplines without first clearing the energy blocks in their physical and emotional bodies. This way of proceeding can cause the equivalent of a short circuit in their systems, as spiritual practices may generate more power than their bodies or minds can handle. Many monks from different Buddhist sects in China have had to seek out Taoist masters to repair the damage to their systems caused by overly forceful meditation techniques. That is why qigong is only a preparatory practice for Taoist meditation. Qigong can help calm an agitated mind and your negative emotions, strengthen the nerves, clear energy blocks and make you healthy.

However, qigong alone is normally insufficient to resolve and clear serious and traumatic emotional and spiritual blockages within the deeper layers of your consciousness. This more encompassing skill primarily belongs in the realm of Taoist meditation.

A Complete System of Personal Development

Qigong represents a total system of energy work. The exercises presented in this book are all that are necessary to maintain high-level health and increase overall awareness. This set of exercises can also serve as warm-up exercises for internal martial artists and energetic healers. These will give the average person at least as much internal benefit as they would most likely obtain from the practice of tai chi with the vast majority of the tai chi teachers in the West, as most teachers either do not know or do not share information regarding the internal energy work of tai chi.

Qigong Can Be Practiced by People of Any Religion

Qigong was primarily developed as an exercise to keep people healthy and reduce tension. Qigong is practiced by people of all spiritual and religious persuasions. Although the basis of qigong is Taoism, one of the primary Eastern religions, there is no necessity to learn or believe its philosophy to practice qigong.

Qigong Is Not a Cult

For five thousand years, Taoists have practiced techniques for developing chi. Most modern Taoists are reluctant to publicly declare that they do qigong and other energy work, preferring to quietly practice in private.

The United States and Europe are presently besieged by cults. Generally speaking, people involved in qigong do their best to avoid cultish identification. Qigong is something you do, something that benefits your life. It is not you, you are not it. However, qigong can have potent effects and some cult groups have incorporated qigong techniques into their practices to draw in adherents. The phenomenon of cults is something China has seen many times and has deemed to be nonessential in terms of human evolution and the development of consciousness.

The Taoists used qigong to make the body healthier, the mind more clear and balanced, the emotions calmer and to increase spiritual capacities. They did not believe in making the practice of qigong yet another wedge to divide people into groups of those who do and those who do not.

The Mind Directs the Chi

The science of qigong is based on the axiom that the mind has the ability to direct chi, which this book can teach you how to accomplish. You can learn to feel your central nervous system, which is a primary intermediary between thoughts and chi. Anyone practicing qigong can begin to feel their nerves, and this ability increases with time. You can literally learn to go inside your body with your mind, feel what is there, and direct your chi where it needs to go. This is not a mysterious process, but a natural one that can be acquired with time and effort.

It is possible to get 50 to 60 percent of the potential health benefits of tai chi just by doing these exercises, which are probably only one-tenth as difficult to learn as tai chi. In addition, there are higher level techniques in tai chi, which are accessible only after mastering all the internal material of these qigong exercises.

Relationship of Qigong to Tai Chi

In the West, most systems of tai chi or other internal martial arts are taught from the viewpoint of movement, with principles such as softness, relaxation, and body alignment thrown in. However, most of the internal components of tai chi that bring about health are commonly overlooked. Whether this lack of information is due to the reticence of teachers or the language and cultural barriers between China and the West, a large vacuum of knowledge does exist for Westerners. This book fills that vacuum.

The traditional and complete internal martial arts of tai chi, hsing-i, and bagua are extremely subtle and advanced forms of qigong. Authentic material on these arts is rarely found in the West and, where it is found, the transmissions tend to be clouded.

Many Benefits to Group Practice of Qigong

As tai chi is often performed in groups, so too, qigong can be done by the young and the old together, to the mutual benefit of both. In Western society at present, young, middle-aged, and elderly people do not spend very much time with each other on a person-to-person basis, without hierarchical constraints. Lack of respect among differing generations is endemic in the United States and Europe. If different age groups continue to avoid spending leisure time together, the tendency toward separation (an "us and them" mentality) will naturally grow.

In China, it is quite common to see a group of about 200 people practicing together, about half over 60 with other ages evenly represented. When people practice qigong, they tap into their inner nature, and after practice it is very common to see the different age groups engaged in friendly conversations, usually related to qigong. Because everyone has been exchanging energy on a subtle level, the barriers between people are easily dissolved, which has kept a generational harmony among qigong groups in China that is virtually unparalleled anywhere else in the world.

The value of qigong, both for the individual and for society, has been proven by millions of people in China, one of the most crowded environments the world has ever known. As such, it could easily meet the needs of the West, with its overcrowded cities and incredible stresses.

Qigong Teaches the Art of Moderation: The 70 Percent Rule

The heart of all Taoist energy practices is the 70 percent rule or rule of moderation. What enables people of all ages to achieve the benefits of qigong and apply them to their everyday life is learning to practice and live with moderation.

The rule states that you should only do a qigong movement, or any chi technique, to approximately 70 percent of your capacity. This is opposite to the "no pain, no gain" principle that is commonly advocated in the West.

Striving for 100 percent produces tension and stress. As soon as you strain or go beyond your capacity, your body has a natural tendency to tense or shut down. Staying within your comfort boundaries will enable your physical and emotional tensions to gradually decrease and, in time, disappear. Although it may seem counterintuitive, the more you relax on every level, the more energy, stamina, range of motion, flexibility and strength you will gain.

These Qigong Exercises Are Safe for All Ages

These exercises are among the most efficient and powerful health maintenance exercises anyone is likely to find. They are gentle, low impact exercises that are easy on the joints and can be done by people who cannot do other forms of aerobic exercise or yoga, and by the sick or injured.

Qigong can do wonders to rejuvenate the elderly. In fact, more than 50 percent of the people who begin tai chi and qigong in China do so after the age of 60, when the realities of aging can no longer be pushed aside. Already, hundreds of millions of people over the age of 60 have found qigong to be uniquely effective. If a form of exercise can make the old functionally younger, its effect on the young or middle-aged is inestimable. If nothing else, it is guaranteed to help release stress, as well as improve your sex life.

These particular qigong exercises can even be adapted for use by the bedridden in hospitals. They are quite safe. Anyone can do them. This is not the case with some types of qigong, which, without the constant supervision of a teacher, may cause significant damage.

The chi flow in the body may be likened to an electrical system. If there is not enough insulation on the wires, or the circuits are connected improperly, the system can short-circuit or otherwise malfunction. Obviously, you do not want this happening to your body.

Although there are hundreds of qigong systems, the techniques they use (which have countless names) can be boiled down to five or six basic types. Some qigong systems require that a teacher meet regularly with no more than a few students at a time in order to prevent potential damage. There are qigong systems that must only be begun before puberty. There are methods that are inappropriate for certain groups to practice, such as males, or females, or people with specific health problems, or people of certain emotional dispositions, or people who have been injured physically or mentally. The exercises presented in this series are the best that could ethically be put in print for the general public, as they can be practiced by almost anyone, which is as safe as any qigong system gets.

The West's Medical Crisis

Until about 1980, the medical systems of the United States and Europe ran reasonably well. Up to that time, the over-60 population fluctuated at somewhere below ten percent of the total population.

As the baby boomers age, the percentage of elderly in the population continues to rise. According to the U.S. Census Bureau, in 1993, one in eight Americans was older than 65; by 2030, the number is expected to be one in five—70 million elderly or 20 percent of the population!

Older people require significantly more medical attention for the same illness than younger people do. For example, a thirty-year old with liver problems, even caused by alcohol, might need a week or two in a hospital. However, a person over sixty could need four to six weeks for the same problem. The deterioration of our medical system is partly due to this simple fact.

According to the Centers for Disease Control and Prevention, chronic diseases are the cause of 70 percent of deaths of our elderly. These are generally life-style diseases that are not caused by infection. They have long, debilitating courses and are rarely cured. These diseases include arthritis, asthma, heart disease, high blood pressure, poor circulation and depression. They are termed life-style diseases because they are caused by living and working in unhealthy environments or by stress, alcohol, tobacco, poor diet or lack of exercise.

Chronic diseases cause great human suffering for the people that have them and for those that love and care for them. Chronic diseases now have a severe impact on the lives of countless children and young adults.

The amount of money spent on doctors, hospital stays and pharmaceuticals to mitigate chronic disease is enormous. For example, arthritis, which limits the activity of over seven million people, is second only to heart disease as a cause of worker disability. By 2020, an estimated 60 million Americans will be affected by arthritis and more than 11 million will be disabled by it. Recent estimates place the direct medical cost of arthritis at $15.2 billion per year, with total costs of medical care and lost wages exceeding $64 billion.

If people take measures to better care for themselves and mitigate stress and arthritis, more health care money will be available for research, infectious disease prevention, surgery, etc.

New ways must be found to enhance and maintain fitness among the elderly. According to the National Center for Health Statistics, Data Warehouse on Trends in Health and Aging, in 1998, 69.2 percent of Medicare beneficiaries sixty-five and over had trouble stooping and 45.6 percent had trouble walking. In 1998, over 30 percent reported having difficulty with heavy housework and about 18 percent reported difficulty with shopping.

Qigong is a great alternative health practice that can help people take control of their well-being, stay healthy and prevent or mitigate chronic illness.

Health Insurance Does Not Guarantee Good Health

Insurance companies keep increasing their rates dramatically, particularly for people over fifty. Moreover, in 2005, one in six people in America did not have health care insurance, and these numbers are expected to get worse.

If the trend continues, people will not be able to afford health insurance unless they are very wealthy.

Basic Questions Regarding the Health Crisis

The statistics speak volumes about the growing costs of health care and the desire of health insurance companies to avoid bearing the burden of those costs.

This leads to some very basic questions, which every Westerner should seriously consider. For example, is my health my responsibility or the responsibility of others? Can I trust my health to insurance companies and HMOs that have excellent financial reasons to make my medical care less than it could be? Will I be denied health care, period? How will I feel if I have to enter a nursing home? Do I genuinely want to be physically and mentally active in my later years, and I am willing to put in the time and effort—through qigong—to achieve this? Am I willing to make a long-term commitment to regularly practicing qigong regularly—or something else that continuously regenerates me—to maintain my health and reduce my stress? Can I stick with something like qigong or tai chi long term, without depending on products or services that promise instant gratification? Can I change my life-style habits to include qigong as a daily practice?

The Qigong Solution to China's Medical Crisis

After the revolution in 1949, China found itself with less than half of its former medical personnel, both Western and traditional. The rest had been killed, fled the country, or gone underground. During the Mao era, the population increased from 400 to 800 million.

The government acknowledged the crisis. Having no interest whatsoever in facing a counter-revolution, leaders took draconian measures. Fortunately, what they implemented worked. The national health problem stabilized until the quantity of medical personnel needed was finally restored.

What the government did was this: they told the top tai chi teachers that they must design tai chi and qigong programs for the health of the general population. Many of these masters wanted to keep their secrets to themselves, so their families could retain their "patents." It has been said that the government insisted that they make their secrets public, or face the extermination of their families down to the last child or relative. Given traditional

Chinese family values, this would have loosened things up significantly, and a national program of tai chi, incorporating many of the principles in this book, was set up across the country.

Non-emergency patients visiting hospitals with complaints from chronic illnesses caused by poor lifestyle or overwork were directed to the hospital administrator. There, they were provided with an ID card and given the name of a nearby tai chi or qigong practitioner. If patients wanted to qualify for another doctor's appointment, or admittance to a hospital, they were required to have their card stamped every day for three months by a local tai chi or qigong instructor, certifying that they had practiced. It must be remembered that the only access to medical care was through the government—there were few, if any, private doctors in China at this time.

The system worked. Tai chi and qigong managed to keep health matters as stable as they could be kept given the poor sanitation and starvation diet most lived with. For the Chinese to get through this incredibly rough period, from the mid 1950s on, it is estimated that between 100 and 200 million people practiced tai chi or qigong daily. Qigong is currently becoming more popular than tai chi in urban environments because available space keeps getting tighter in China, and qigong requires less of it.

Tai chi and qigong are the only internal energy systems that have actually been practiced by and have worked for large masses of a population. Yoga practitioners never exceeded one percent of India's population. Considering the parallels between the problems presented by the West's aging population and what China went through, it is encouraging that qigong methods can serve as a model for preventing a great deal of the medical misery that our increased elderly population will most certainly be confronting. Socialized medicine alone is not the answer; many European countries with socialized medicine are facing the same problems. Aging populations that require high-tech medical care simply create too much expense to bear.

The Benefits of Qigong

Loosens the Muscles and Builds Power

Qigong works with the muscles quite differently than the typical exercises practiced by Westerners. Aerobics and vigorous stretching build strength and flexibility; qigong and other internal exercises build effortless power and looseness. The feeling of strength, of being "pumped up," obtained in Western exercise is actually due to muscular contraction, that prevents the free flow of chi, even though such exercise may give you the extreme flexibility to be able to do leg splits, for example.

In the internal arts, the feeling of muscular strength is considered inappropriate; the goal, rather, is a feeling of relaxed power. Relaxed power comes when the muscles, rather than fighting and straining to do something, just loosen (open up) and allow the energy to flow through.

Strengthens the Organs

The qigong techniques discussed in this book—especially the three swings—work to strengthen and balance all the internal organs. There are also other techniques (not mentioned in this book) to strengthen specific organs: to help the liver recover from hepatitis, for instance, or the lungs from tuberculosis, or the heart from a heart attack. Even without having had a serious illness, almost everyone is born with a weakness in one organ or another, and qigong has precise exercises to address an individual's specific problems.

Improves Cardio-pulmonary Function

Most people think that aerobic exercise is necessary to strengthen the heart and lungs. While aerobic exercise does accomplish this, so does qigong. Slow, deep, regular breathing and energy movement combine to work oxygen deeper into the tissues than regular exercise.

One case in point: a qigong student who holds a normal, sedentary office job and engages in almost no aerobic activity has a brother who is a well-known mountaineer. Invited to climb a mountain in Colorado with his brother, he imagined himself gasping for air as his brother marched ahead, but much to his surprise he found that his capacity for physical activity, in terms of breath, had actually come to surpass that of his brother, who engaged in aerobic activity continuously.

Strengthens the Nerves

A primary way chi flows is along the nerves of the body. Although at advanced levels of development chi and the nerves can be felt separately, the great majority of beginners only have an awareness of their nerves.

The nerves are an intermediary between the body and the mind, and it is through the nerves that we can gain access to information about our body. Much of the initial qigong work, which emphasizes getting in touch with the body and clearing out blockages, is accomplished through the nervous system. As your chi gets stronger through continued practice, your nerves are strengthened and your body awareness is enhanced. People with poor coordination and other motor problems can benefit greatly. The spinal nerves play a vital role in overall health. Indeed, the entire chiropractic system is based on the importance of spinal nerve flow.

Like the nerves, chi is also an intermediary between the body and the mind, and while it travels with nerve impulses, it can, with practice, be felt independently. It is commonly said in the internal arts that the mind moves the chi, and the chi moves the body. While this is true, it is important to be aware that most beginners need to work through the nerves first.

Qigong's ability to strengthen the nervous system makes it a magnificently effective technique for relieving stress on a day-to-day basis, as well as rebuilding bodies that have broken down due to long-term stress.

Improves Vascular Function

Western aerobics increase circulation by exercising the heart. Qigong improves circulation by increasing the elasticity of the blood vessels themselves. It is standard in China to prescribe qigong exercises for both high and low blood pressure, as both are due to problems in vascular elasticity and strength.

Qigong Can Be Used by the Seriously Ill

Western exercise utilizes either motion or resistance to motion to strengthen the body (for example, weight training, calisthenics, running). Unfortunately, the seriously ill and bedridden often do not have the capacity for vigorous exercise. This means that the muscles and organ systems get weaker during prolonged bed rest, and it may take months to get back to normal after recovery from the main problem (a back injury, for instance). Qigong, however, has many techniques specifically designed for the weak and immobile, techniques which increase physical capacities without requiring movement.

In China, qigong is also prescribed for terminally ill cancer patients as a last resort. If they don't initially have the strength to practice while standing or sitting, they can practice lying down until their strength builds up.

Helps Prevent Injury to Joints, Ligaments and Bones

Accidental injury can occur in many ways and joints and ligaments are particularly vulnerable. People habitually lock their joints when falls or accidents occur, and a locked joint is an easily broken joint. Ligaments can easily be overstretched in an accident and getting them to bounce back is very difficult.

Qigong teaches better balance; it also teaches how to turn correctly without straining, to move your joints without locking them and how to relax during a fall. Qigong increases flexibility and the spring of ligaments. Qigong is like a good gentle stretch and an acupuncture treatment combined, which improves the circulation of fluids and energy in the body to lessen the impact of injuries and allow more rapid healing.

Practitioners of qigong learn to avoid strain and stay well within their 70 percent capacity, and, in particular, not to overstrain if there is already some pain or restriction.

Qigong balances energy and improves the weaker areas in people's internal systems. The aim is to prevent the body's "weak links" from causing problems down the road.

Speeds Recovery Time from Injuries and Operations

The gentle, non-jarring and low-impact movements of qigong can be done immediately following an injury or operation, particularly if the 70 percent rule is adhered to and no strain is applied. This rule is particularly important during healing, as the body is already overstressed.

First, parts of the body that were not injured can be gently moved and exercised. These movements will increase the circulation of bodily fluids and the flow of energy to all parts of the body. The lymph system will be energized, which helps to improve the immune system. Opening the energy channels will enable the natural healing abilities of the body to accelerate rapidly.

Second, qigong helps the entire body and mind to relax. During injuries, the body and mind tense. Tension in the uninjured areas of the body will suck up chi necessary to heal the injured parts. Qigong helps to relax the parts of the body that were not injured. This gradually takes tension out of the body to help the body heal faster. Doing something proactive and effective to speed recovery also can diminish anger and fear.

Applying the rule of no strain helps injuries to heal fully. The 70 percent rule allows recovery to happen gradually and fully. Injuries that are only partially resolved can progressively weaken other parts of the body and set up conditions for major problems in uninjured areas, immediately or over time.

Builds Athletic and Martial Arts Power

Qigong is the basis of the power of the Chinese martial arts, whether kung fu, or the more subtle internal forms, such as tai chi, hsing-i, and bagua. It is almost impossible to determine from an external view how the seemingly gentle, smooth movements of the internal forms enable the advanced practitioner to defeat the most violent street fighter. This capability is basically derived from the practice of qigong, which develops chi and internal power.

People who train in the internal martial arts will find that practicing the material revealed in this book will enable them to surpass inherent physical strength and athletic abilities.

Eases Stress and Balances Emotions

Much of the new literature on stress indicates that one of the largest factors in determining stress levels is the emotions. Most physical exercise is at least somewhat useful for relieving anger, but one need only look at the behavior of some top athletes to see that typical physical activity does not necessarily balance the emotions.

The clearing process in qigong can be used on strongly repressed, as well as on spontaneously over-expressed emotions. Many of the movements of qigong can be refined to specifically address your problem area, be it depression, grief, frustration, irritability, or any combination thereof.

Stress-related problems in our society are worsening, so it is urgent to gain the ability to convert the energy of negative and destructive emotions to those that are more positive in nature. The ability to release stress directly through control of the central nervous system is a method par excellence for dealing with burnout.

Benefits Sedentary Workers and Meditators

Sitting too long can weaken your body. The circulation of your fluids becomes sluggish and your tension increases. This strains your nervous system, which lessens the ability of your mind to remain fully awake and concentrate on meditation or prayers.

A classic story handed down from the sixth century is that a Buddhist master came to China's Shaolin Temple, which became the home of Chan Buddhism. He found that the monks would easily become distracted and would even fall asleep during meditation. He realized that their sincerity was genuine but their energy was not always up to the task. The Buddhist master taught the monks a form of qigong that later became the basis of China's Shaolin qigong school. Chan Buddhism was later taken to Japan and became the foundation for Zen Buddhism.

The purpose of teaching monks qigong was to provide them with a stable internal body and energy structure to keep them physically comfortable and mentally alert. Qigong enabled them to sit cross-legged on the floor comfortably for prolonged periods, without stiffness, pain or loss of energy.

The qigong exercises in this book can do the same for anyone engaged in long periods of prayer or meditation, whether sitting on the floor or in a chair.

In the same way, these exercises will help anyone in a sedentary job to be better able to concentrate and stay comfortable when sitting at a desk or computer for hours at a time.

Mette Heinz

Bruce Frantzis works with a student on the alignments of the Second Swing of Opening the Energy Gates of Your Body Qigong. Practicing this exercise with correct alignments loosens tension in the joints, ligaments and internal organs.

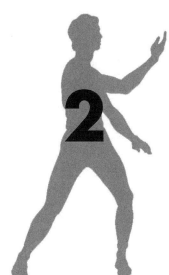

2 How Qigong Works

The Internal Mechanics: Qigong and Body Health

Qigong works strongly on the body fluids, including blood, lymph, and the synovial and cerebrospinal fluids.

Blood Is Circulated Without Stress on the Heart

Unlike aerobics, qigong does not dramatically increase the heart rate during exercise. The object of qigong is not to make the heart pump more strongly, but to increase the elasticity of the vascular system. As the vessels expand and contract with more vigor, the heart does not need to pump as strongly, thereby providing it with more rest. Thus, the beneficial consequences of qigong and internal martial arts are primarily vascular in nature.

The Lymph Pump and Immune System Are Strengthened

The lymph fluids are moved primarily by tiny muscular expansions and contractions. The qigong techniques taught here employ some of their strongest motions where the largest lymph nodes are located; that is, the armpits, the backs of the knees, and the inguinal region. Qigong's relatively fine muscular expansions and contractions move lymph efficiently through the entire system. These actions, as well as the overall increase in chi that qigong brings, strengthen the body's immune response.

Synovial Fluid Is Revitalized, Bringing Flexibility to Joints

Synovial fluid is found in joints. It lubricates them, allows joint flexibility, and when functioning normally, helps prevent arthritis and rheumatism. From the point of view of Chinese medicine, when "wind/damp" or physical obstructions (coagulated blood, calcium deposits, and so on) get struck in the joints, the results are not only specific joint problems but a decrease in the flow of chi through the entire body as well. Qigong works with the synovial fluid by compressing and expanding it, preventing and reversing all sorts of joint problems.

Cerebrospinal Pump Becomes Efficient

Cerebrospinal fluid is basically a nutrient bath and lubricating liquid that surrounds the spinal cord and brain. It keeps a constant pressure in the human body, which regulates nerve flow and affects every physical sense. The quality of your physical senses is determined by the health of your spine. Your cerebrospinal fluid, to a great degree, determines just how healthy your spinal cord is and how efficiently the spinal nerves carry messages from your brain to your body and from your body to your brain. All qigong work strongly affects the cerebrospinal pump, both by physically pumping fluid and by moving chi, all of which encourages the spine to perform at optimal efficiency.

Muscle Tissue Gains Elasticity

Qigong also causes muscle tissue to elongate. This activity differs from stretching in the usual sense. The object here is to fill the tissues with energy, so that they stabilize at a given degree of stretch. With most forms of stretching, the body soon shrinks back to its original state when the stretch stops. With the stretches of qigong, however, the muscles eventually attain a state similar to that of a springy rubber band. A few athletes possess this muscular springiness naturally, but anyone can attain this state with qigong practice.

Tendons Are Strengthened

Qigong also adds greater strength and elasticity to the tendons. This contributes to the tremendous flexibility and physical power many qigong practitioners have, which derives primarily from the tendons and ligaments, not from the muscles. Qigong has the ability to not only make ligaments more springy but also to shrink and stabilize overstretched ligaments, which make a joint too floppy—a problem experienced by many dancers.

Bone Marrow Is Energized

Qigong affects the bones by directly infusing the bone marrow with energy. This technique is an advanced one, but by the time a disciplined practitioner reaches an advanced level of qigong, the energizing of the bone marrow has started to occur.

Body Cells Are Healed

Masters of qigong have been healing people suffering from chronic or incurable diseases since ancient times. In China today, there are sections of hospitals and clinics that use qigong to treat conditions unresponsive to other methods of therapy, such as Western medicine, acupuncture and herbs. Here patients learn to regulate their own chi, with a little help from their therapist. The range of maladies amenable to such treatment is quite broad, ranging from nerve diseases, such as Parkinson's, to cellular diseases, such as cancer.

The Process of Awakening Chi

Your body will awaken in stages. If you constantly practice qigong, your body will open up in layers. Muscles that were initially numb will begin to regain sensation. Your body will reveal itself to you gradually, in a marvelous process of discovery. As your body becomes more alive you will be able to feel how your physical self works from the inside out.

It is not farfetched to say that you may actually begin to feel your internal organs, for example, kinesthetically sense where your liver and spleen are, and what they are doing at any given time, as opposed to knowing this information only intellectually. This sensitivity allows for detecting potential problems well before they ever get to the point of causing trouble.

The Body-Awakening Process Is Irregular

The process of opening the body is more often like an uneven roller coaster than a linear journey. One week one part of your body will open; the next week another part will open, while a previously open part closes again. The process is a bit like a game of "now you see it, now you don't." The time will come, though, when your body will open up and stay open, completely accessible to your awareness.

Never Force Open Body Parts That Are Blocked

What happens if you encounter, and cannot get rid of, a particular block during standing qigong or some other exercise? The answer is simple: Do not force it. Rather than remaining at that one unmovable block and working away at it fruitlessly for a prolonged time, just move on to the next step. You may find that the next day or week the immovable block will quite suddenly dissolve.

Your Chi Is Growing Even if You Cannot Feel It

What happens if you practice qigong for a while but do not feel anything different happening in your body? This is, in fact, the case for many people. It takes time for you to become sensitive to chi, but a good rule of thumb to go by is as follows: If you find yourself feeling more comfortable, or if you are able to do more things without strain, or if you do not get sick as often as you used to, or if you start developing a type of effortless concentration and ability to do physical activities you never before even thought were possible—your chi is growing whether you are aware of it or not. Keep practicing and you will eventually feel the chi in a very real, direct way.

Strange Sensations Are Normal

Some of the common sensations people report when they feel the chi starting to move in their bodies include: feelings of warmth, extreme heat, electricity, heaviness, lightness, expansion, contraction, pressure, and internal sense of wind or water moving.

Qigong Frees Trapped Emotions

When energy enters your system it affects every level of your being. Some of its physical effects have already been mentioned. However, as the chi grows stronger in the body, it also charges up emotional energies.

Large numbers of people in the West are very repressed emotionally, as they have spent a great deal of time and effort learning to control their emotions. Emotions that have never been expressed stay in the energy body of a human being at the fringes of conscious awareness. As you open up the chi flow in your system, the chi can give emotional energy more power, just as it strengthens your physical energy.

Increased emotional energy enables you to feel your present emotions, as well as those you have suppressed for a long period of time. Emotions such as anger, fear, love, hate, sadness, or joy may arise for no apparent reason. Often during practice, or more commonly a few hours after, such feelings, stronger in nature, may suddenly appear. It is important to understand that these sensations, which we call emotions, do not require acting upon—just quietly experience them internally and let them wash through you.

If a person feels angry and takes it out on someone else, either physically or mentally, the anger many actually increase rather than be dispelled. On the other hand, if the dissolving techniques taught in this book are used on the "emotional body," (see p. 51, "Neigong and The Energy Bodies") that same anger can be transformed into a healthy, usable form. Behaviorally acting out negative emotional energy that was stuck to begin with may only further entrench it. Again, understand that nothing has to be "done" with this energy. You can merely observe it, monitoring it as it dissolves and is re-assimilated and ultimately transformed into a healthy constructive force. On the energetic level, it is just as unhealthy to throw excessive emotional energy around externally as it is to repress it.

Taoist, Kundalini and Western Psychotherapy

The Taoist view of the transformation of emotional energy differs radically from the cathartic practices of either Eastern kundalini or Western group therapy. In the Shaktipat kundalini practice, catharsis is sometimes called *kriya*, or action. Here, the idea, in the early developmental stages, is to discharge emotional energy by various actions, such as screaming, yelling, crying, curling into the fetal position—moving through blocked emotional states until they are freed up. In group therapy (from primal scream to encounter, bioenergetics, and psychodrama) the idea is to emote your pain and agony externally, the louder the better, heaping verbal and physical abuse on a pillow or a person, as the case may be. Though these approaches are sometimes successful, the ancient Taoists detected an inherent problem with such techniques.

When pressure builds up in a pressure cooker, there are—within the cathartic model—only three options you have to handle the situation: 1) turn the heat off (i.e., deny, repress); 2) let some steam out at intervals; or 3) let all the steam out at once. Turning the heat off leaves the basic emotional situation unchanged. If you only let steam partially out, after a period, the pressure will build to again reach a critical level. All the "steam" can be let out of a trapped emotion at one blow, but the reality is that this particular event rarely occurs. Far more common for people with emotional blockages is that they let some, but not all, of the emotional pressure out, and then—as mentioned—the pressure rebuilds until they have to "cathart" again.

The cathartic release of violent emotions irritates and exhausts the system, and can sometimes foster an addictive need to feel those violent emotions in ever-stronger forms. Cathartic methods may easily turn practitioners into therapy junkies—angry people become angrier still, for instance, or depressed people sink deeper into depression, while deluding themselves into thinking that they are working on self-improvement.

Taoist Therapy Emphasizes Dissolving Emotions into the Flow of Chi

The Taoists found that emotional energy can be manipulated more or less like physical energy. Thus, Taoist practices are based on allowing emotional energy to move through your system until it completes itself; there is no attempt to push the energy out or to prevent it from occurring in the first place. The principles are quite similar to what one finds in acupuncture. In acupuncture, when a needle is first inserted into a point in the body, the needle may vibrate as it encounters blocked energy. When this blocked energy finally breaks through and continues moving on its path, the needle then stops shaking. It does not matter how powerful the energy going through the line (or meridian) is; what is important is whether or not it gets stopped or blocked.

Therefore, simply let the emotional energy that comes up find its way through your system. If the emotions are too strong for you to handle, follow the same pattern suggested for dealing with a block in the physical body; namely, back off and try to dissolve the block again later, so that it diminishes slowly over time. Attempting to resolve the situation in one great extremist heroic effort will not work, and may cause a lot of unnecessary misery.

Emotions are only sensations, which we then designate as good or bad. The sensations themselves are fairly neutral. Qigong practitioners learn to differentiate between frequencies of energy that are intrinsically benevolent to their emotions (but nonetheless can evoke thoughts, even uncomfortable ones, that have to be dealt with) and energy running through the emotional body that is essentially malevolent; that is, destructive to the overall energy system.

The arousal of emotional issues during the practice of qigong is a positive sign. It is far better to move through old emotional blocks than to go through life emotionally shut down. It is significantly healthier to learn to dissolve, on a daily basis, the negative emotions you are constantly exposed to than absorb them and then abuse your spouse, child, dog, or anyone else who happens to be around you.

It is my hope that the emotional-release function of qigong, almost unknown in the West, becomes common knowledge. It is extraordinarily powerful, humane and gentle, and could prove of great value in the Western world. Qigong for emotional energy transformation is not dramatic, just effective.

Qigong Does Not Replace Psychotherapy or Medical Advice

The effect of qigong practice on those with severe psychological or emotional problems is unpredictable. These people should not practice qigong without being monitored by an appropriate health care professional. In the East, sometimes people with these problems may be able to go to ashrams or monasteries, where their practice can be closely monitored and adjusted as necessary to work towards a successful outcome. Such facilities are rarely found in the West.

Cultivate Your Chi Slowly and Safely

All safe chi development practices are cumulative and progress slowly, developing strong links between the brain and the chi. In this context, "strong" refers to the ability of the nerves to convey messages between the mind and the chi clearly, with sufficient "insulation" and "resistance" to avoid burnout. A strong nervous system allows messages to be delivered between the brain and the chi without conscious will or effort. Until the nerves have been developed, the will must be used to transmit messages, much as a baby at first has to use tremendous will power to crawl and walk until the appropriate nerve pathways between the brain and the chi are forged. Once those links are in place, you do not need to think about walking, you simply walk.

The development of chi must of necessity be slow and steady in order for it to be stable. Once this is understood, it is easy to see how the incorrect practice of qigong can lead to problems. Appendix C talks about this issue.

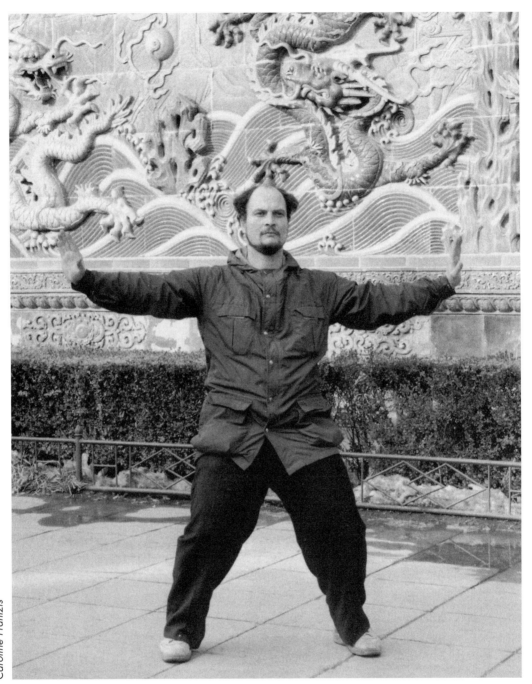

Caroline Frantzis

Bruce Frantzis demonstrates one of the 200 or so qigong standing postures at the Nine Dragon Wall in Beijing, China, in the winter of 1986. See Chapter 15 for more details on standing postures.

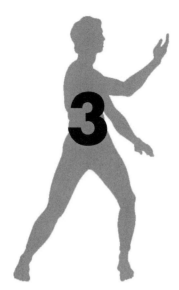

3 Qigong Theory

The Gap Between Qigong as It Is Taught in China and the West

I returned to the West in 1987, after more than a decade of intense study of the internal arts in China. Since then, I have conducted workshops, retreats and instructor trainings attended by many tai chi and qigong students and teachers, who had anywhere from one to twenty years of experience. It has been my observation that many of the most fundamental (and essential) principles of tai chi and qigong have never been explained to these individuals, many of whom are now, or will be, teachers of these arts.

In fact, at the present time, much of the Western practice of the internal arts (tai chi chuan, qigong, hsing-i chuan and bagua zhang) is based solely on physical movements and mental visualizations. Many students only imitate the external movements of their teachers, believing that this type of practice will increase their flow of chi, thereby giving them power and health. These students have to guess at what their teachers are doing internally, with no way of knowing if their guesses are correct.

The Chinese Language Barrier

Other students whom I have taught did receive explanations about internal energy from their Chinese teachers; unfortunately the information imparted was not always accurate, as their teachers often did not speak English well and translators lacked sufficient knowledge to translate this highly technical subject into English. Vague generalities were often substituted for specific information. In many cases, the problem was the original teacher's sheer unwillingness to transmit the specific training methodologies clearly.

In the process of transferring wisdom from one culture to another, difficulties and common misunderstandings are the rule rather than the exception. Tai chi and qigong have been known in the West since the 1960s and now the time has come to help clear up people's misconceptions about these arts.

A majority of the early translators were not themselves expert in the fields of tai chi and qigong. Consequently, metaphorical descriptions were commonly mistaken for actual methods of practice. As in any specialized field, technical terms can have radically different meanings and connotations for insiders. The general public may be familiar with the words themselves, but ignorant of their precise intent. Since most people with expertise in the field of chi development are Chinese, metaphors in the Chinese language are used to describe what adepts are doing. These metaphors make perfect sense from an Oriental perspective, but often lead Westerners down the wrong path.

As much as possible, this chapter will try to demystify and clarify the common cross-cultural confusion inherent in this area and, more importantly, convey in English the processes that are involved in the basic practices of these internal arts.

The Challenge of Transplanting Chinese Cultural Ideas

After I became truly bilingual, I noticed that even when I was processing the same information in my mind, I would think and feel quite differently in each language. This happens because the cultural and linguistic context in which people learn to view life determines to a great extent what they feel, and how they think information should be communicated. This cultural matrix dictates not only what should remain unstated but also how what is left unsaid should be interpreted.

These issues have caused great difficulties in communicating the subjects of tai chi and qigong to Westerners. The Chinese leave much unsaid, assuming that much of what is relegated to silence anybody (meaning anyone with an average Chinese education) would understand. Unfortunately, the Chinese cultural background contains information that most Westerns have no access to. Here are some basic definitions.

Traditional Qigong and Neigong: What's the Difference?

Before the 1950s, the term *qigong* was rarely used in China for chi development practices; the more prevailing terms were *neigong* (internal power) and *lien gong* (practice power). During the second half of the twentieth century, however, the term qigong gained ascendancy, especially in mainland China, where one finds a variety of forms, many with poetic or strange names, such as White Crane Qigong, Old Man Climbs the Stairs Qigong, Plum Blossom Qigong, and so forth.

All qigong practices are derived from the parent neigong systems. The techniques found in this volume, for example, are all original neigong practices.[1] The 16 components of the neigong system and their relationship to the core exercises of this book are described in Chapter 15.

These energy systems were discovered and developed by Taoist monks as they delved deeply into their minds and bodies during meditation. They used chi energy to maintain superior health, heal illness and realize profound inner stillness and spirituality. Their work was codified as the neigong system, which formed the energetic foundation of qigong—the internal martial arts of tai chi, hsing-i and bagua; Taoist healing arts, including acupuncture and qigong tui na; and Taoist meditation.

These ancient methods, which have been kept relatively secret for millennia, have immense depth. A good teacher can communicate neigong techniques from beginning to the more advanced levels. Appendix B includes instructions for finding a qualified teacher.

Neigong Moves from the Inside Out; Qigong Moves from the Outside In

The emphasis in neigong is on developing the core energy that travels through the center of the body, and, from the core, opening and energizing the peripheral energy lines such as the acupuncture meridians. Qigong concentrates on working the more superficial energy lines first, and, through these, indirectly affecting the core energy. In this sense, qigong is similar to acupuncture, which also manipulates the more superficial and peripheral energy through the meridians, collateral channels and eight special meridians to bring about changes at a deeper level.

---

[1] Throughout this book, the author uses the expression qigong, because it has become a blanket term, a kind of brand name, in the West. However, the material in this book involves neigong practices rather than the more limited perspective upon which many modern qigong systems are based.

Qigong Moves Chi with Separate Body Movements; Neigong Moves Chi through Multiple Simultaneous Mind-Body Interactions

In qigong, the practitioner works one chi technique at a time, combining them gradually into a specific sequence. For instance, in one physical movement, one acupuncture channel is opened, then, once opened, the practitioner opens the next in line with a different physical movement, and so on. Various techniques are used in qigong, from slapping to stretching to stomping, but the most important principle to remember about qigong in general is that one separate chi flow is sequentially followed by another. Two or more rarely go on simultaneously.

Qigong in general tends to focus on specific acupuncture channels and points, whereas neigong is likely to work more with the energy of the central channel (see energy anatomy diagram on p. 239)—which runs from the crown of the head to the perineum and through the center of the bones of the arms and legs—as well as with the muscles, fascia, internal organs, glands, spinal cord and brain. From a medical perspective, qigong usually utilizes specific techniques for specific problems, while neigong energizes the whole system. This overall improvement in energy function leads to the eventual resolution of particular problems.

The neigong system seeks to work all the chi flows of the system at one time, the ultimate objective being to synergistically combine the hundreds of chi flows in the body within every movement. This way, the practitioner will eventually have access to energy, which, in its totality, is more than just the sum of the chi flowing through the channels. At high levels, the chi of the body, mind and spirit integrates. The whole person then functions like a single huge cell, with all its chi pulsing in unison.

Although neigong is learned one piece at a time, it should always be practiced in a way that all learned pieces are performed simultaneously. Eventually, the practitioner's energy permeates to the center of both the bone marrow and the spine. For this reason, neigong is generally considered superior for people who want to have both a high level of health and great physical prowess.

Put simply, the main difference between qigong and neigong is that, in qigong, technique A is followed by technique B followed by technique C; the effect of these is the cumulative effect of A plus B plus C. With neigong, however, technique A is done at the same time as B and C; the effect is that of A multiplied by B multiplied by C.

In Qigong, the Breath Moves the Chi Indirectly; In Neigong, the Mind Moves the Chi Directly

In the Chinese internal arts, the term "breath" refers to two distinct processes: first, the movement of the air in and out of the lungs—the physical breath—and second, the ebb and flow of the chi or life force throughout the body—the subtle breath of chi. The physical breath and the subtle breath can be coordinated, or they can work independently. Qigong coordinates the two, while neigong can work directly with the subtle breath only, without depending upon the intermediary of the physical breath.

In qigong, the physical breath is used to forge a link between the mind and the chi or subtle breath. The mind or awareness focuses on the physical breath: you visualize the physical breath moving chi through your body and potentially feel the breath go into a particular part of your body. It thus indirectly makes contact with the chi or subtle breath. The inhales and exhales, suspension, and quickening and slowing of the physical breath are coordinated with whatever you are doing, whether it be body movement, energy development or visualization of the emotional, psychic, or spiritual aspects of your being.

Most Chinese medical qigong methods are based on the use of the physical breath to activate the chi. Similarly, most Buddhist qigong practices are based on awareness of the physical breath. For example, Gautama the Buddha's essential practice, today know as Vipassana, was based upon observing the rise and fall of the physical breath and the sensations in the body. Tantric Buddhism, in its completion stage practices, uses the rhythm of the physical breath as a coordinating medium for mantras, energy work and visualizations.

In neigong, however, the mind or awareness moves the chi directly, with or without the assistance of physical breath. The mind may remain purely aware of the internal energy, or may direct it to specific tasks and energy channels. Neigong uses efficient physical breathing mechanisms that recreate how a baby breathes in the womb, but chi movement is independent of the physical breath, regardless of how you are breathing. The physical breath may sometimes become so slow, quiet, and still as to seem to disappear. Over time, the context of the subtle breath shifts from the physical breath to the presence of the chi or mind itself.

Neigong and the Energy Bodies

For a person doing chi development that involves physical movement, neigong has one inherent advantage over qigong. This advantage relates to the subconscious mind.

In neigong, one works directly with the chi, bypassing, at the beginning levels, the use of the breath to move the chi. The practitioner slowly over time becomes sensitive to how the subtle breath or chi is not only penetrating the physical body, but also the more subtle energy bodies—the emotional body, the mental body, psychic body, the causal body, and so on.[2] Once the connection between the mind and the various chi bodies has been stabilized, one will be aware of how the coordination of the breath with physical and chi movement affects all levels of one's being. Practitioners will then be able to use all aspects of the breath consciously to develop all of their energy bodies equally. They will become aware of the dark, dead emotional spots that need to be dissolved, as well as the bright, alive spots that should be energized. At this more advanced stage, the use of the breath will allow one to strengthen the whole energy body in a strong and balanced way.

Qigong and Neigong Each Have Unique Strengths

Generally, a true neigong expert will understand the methodologies of qigong. However, the reverse is not true—a qigong expert will usually not be aware of all the neigong methods. This would lead one to believe that neigong is superior to qigong, which is not necessarily the case. Many diseases and dysfunctions may be caused by an imbalance in only a small part of a person's system. In these cases, it is best to use qigong techniques because only a limited number of chi flows need to be learned and practiced to address the problem. Neigong is usually more advantageous for longevity and high performance.

The Internal Martial Arts: Tai Chi, Hsing-I and Bagua

The three internal martial arts of tai chi chuan, hsing-i chuan and bagua zhang are all based on the neigong system of chi development. They combine the most effective fighting techniques of ancient China and fuse them with the neigong system of internal power development. This combination produces two seemingly unrelated results: superior competitive athletic and fighting skills and superior health. Tai chi and bagua can, with specific training at high levels, be complete spiritual development systems.

---

2 For more information on the eight energies bodies, see *Relaxing Into Your Being*, by Bruce Frantzis (North Atlantic Books, 2001), Chapter 2.

Tai Chi Is Primarily Practiced for Health in China

In modern China, almost all the people who practice tai chi do so purely to enhance their health, reduce stress, and improve their overall levels of energy. Relatively few of them use it as a martial art, where the increased internal power is utilized to improve fighting ability, whether for attacking, defending, hitting, or absorbing blows. It should be stressed that the training for martial applications is appreciably more rigorous than that for health. Jogging a mile or two a day may be good for health, but to become a marathoner requires significantly more effort. Similarly, practicing tai chi for only 20 to 40 minutes a day can greatly improve well-being, and extend vibrant health into old age. However, training many hours a day and with a highly skilled master for approxmately for ten years is required to become an effective martial artist. To use tai chi to become spiritually realized requires even more effort than martial arts training.

Hsing-I and Bagua: Fighting Methods
That Promote Long Life

Hsing-i is an extremely powerful neigong system, and has been the main internal system used on battlefields in China for the past nine hundred years. Invented by a general who then taught it to his officer corps, hsing-i, in the nineteenth century, became famous as the martial art of convoy guards. It can be considered to be like karate with a great emphasis on developing internal strength and power, as well as producing health.

Hsing-i places great emphasis on developing demonstrable power. While a tai chi master's body becomes soft on the outside and hard on the inside, hsing-i masters seek just the opposite. The outside becomes like a piece of steel and the inside becomes very soft, which leads to incredible physical flexibility as well as a sense of internal comfort. Of the three internal martial arts, hsing-i brings a sense of strength and vitality the most quickly.

Bagua is generally considered to be the highest of the internal martial arts.Both bagua and hsing-i masters tend to live longer than tai chi masters. Bagua practices are more difficult than those of tai chi. In China, they say that everybody can do tai chi, but only a few can do hsing-i and fewer still bagua. Tai chi and hsing-i use circles, but bagua is unique in its use of spheres. Bagua works the energy of the body in such a way that it eventually creates more physical and energetic flexibility than either of the other two internal arts. It is also the most physically beautiful, with its continually manifesting spiraling energy.

While bagua is a very effective martial art, this is but one of its aspects. Based on the internal alchemy energy principles of the *I Ching*, or *Book of Changes*, bagua is a physical method of embodying and manifesting the *I Ching's* energies. It is a sad fact that the genuine energy tradition of bagua is being lost in China and the West. Mostly what one can find now of bagua consists of a series of physical movements or simple martial art applications used in diverse martial art schools. It is very difficult to locate substantial information about the genuine bagua system.

Bagua is the only martial art in China that is completely Taoist in nature, as both tai chi and hsing-i were influenced by the Buddhist Shaolin Monastery. Bagua only became public in the late 1800s, though there is a Taoist monastery in southern China that has been practicing the basic bagua walk for 1,500 years, and they have records of it coming 4,000 years ago from somewhere in the Kunlun mountains. No one really knows how old it is.

The practice sets of all three internal martial arts are composed of a series of postures that are done in sequences of movements. (For a definition of "posture" as used in Taoist energy arts, see p. 235.) In the fashion of all neigong practices, each of the postures works with all the body's chi flows simultaneously. Each posture has one major energetic function and the entire set of consecutive interlinked postures develops a specific energetic quality. The goal of these movements is to clear blockages, making the overall chi in the body more powerful and balanced.

The same life energy developed and used by martial artists can also be used by athletes or dancers, enabling them to develop a reserve of inner power that normally only the most talented of champions ever acquire. The difference is that, in the West, athletes find this inner power by accident or birth, whereas the Chinese have found many deliberate, systematic ways of developing this internal power for those willing to take the time to practice consistently.

Three Levels of Qigong: Body, Chi and Mind

The internal methodologies of tai chi chuan, hsing-i and bagua, as well as qigong and neigong, all operate on the three levels of body, chi, and mind/spirit.

The core exercises presented in this volume deal mainly with body and chi development. Their primary focus is not on emptying the mind and attaining stillness and union with the

Tao, which are goals of higher-level meditation and mind development techniques. Before running, one must first learn to stand and walk.

The core exercises herein can have a dual function: 1) You can do them independently, as a form of qigong, even if you know nothing about tai chi. Such practice will provide you with many of the basic health and stress-management benefits that motivate most people to begin tai chi or other internal martial arts in the first place. 2) If you are already involved in the internal martial arts or in sitting meditation, you can do these exercises as warm-ups, so that your body is fully prepared for practice. This reduces the possibility of injuries and dissipates the initial layer of stress that would otherwise have to be resolved during the first half hour of your regular practice. You are thereby free to concentrate on the deeper elements of tai chi or Taoist meditation.

Body Synergy Increases Your Reservoir of Chi

The primary idea behind these core exercises, and, for that matter, behind tai chi and neigong in general, is synergy, meaning that the whole can be more than the sum of the parts. In human activity, synergy is verified experientially. You have to feel it to know whether or not it works. Hundreds of millions of people throughout the centuries in China, and many people in the West, have found that using energy synergistically is of great value.

Simply put, synergy in the core exercises involves coordinating the many elements of body, mind, and energy so that they move simultaneously. For example, if five parts of your body, each having an arbitrary value of two, were to work separately or consecutively, as they would for most people, the resulting energy would be equal to the sum of the parts, or 10 units. Using the parts synergistically would be like multiplying the energy values of the parts, rather than just adding them, and the energy output would ideally equal 32 units.

All of these exercises are performed with the intention of strengthening the central nervous system and the internal organs, rather than only the muscles. Through the application of total relaxation, they first seek to rid the body of accumulated stress and tension. Next, they strengthen the internal organs and nerves of the body, as much as the practitioner's capacity allows. When this capacity is reached, they then increase reserves of chi that can be drawn on naturally in times of stress or emergency.

From the perspective of chi development, many exercises done in the West have a tendency to deplete the body's essential core reserves, mainly because they are so performance-oriented. The competition may be won today, but ten or fifteen years down the road, when deep reserve energy is needed to fight off internal organ problems or cancer, it will not be there. As the adage goes, "follies of youth are paid for in old age."

Importance of Preserving Your "Life Capital"

Qigong practitioners in China believe that a person is born with a certain amount of life energy capital. Let's say most people come into the world with a million dollars, though some rare individuals may be born with hundreds of millions of dollars. For babies, the difference isn't that great between having capital of a million dollars or a hundred million dollars—almost all babies are relaxed, amazingly energetic, and able to recover from illness or injury quickly and easily. It is like a very rich man who is not much affected economically whether he eats at McDonalds or the Ritz—for him, there is not much difference between two dollars and two hundred dollars. The multimillionaires, because of their tremendous genetic good fortune, can smoke three packs of cigarettes and drink two bottles of whisky a day, cavort into the late hours of the night, get next to no sleep, work inhumanely long hours, and still live to be ninety-five years old without serious illness. For the other 99.9 percent of the population, however, a lifestyle like this would cause great misery and an early demise.

Major illnesses, injuries or surgeries deplete one's life-energy capital significantly. One either makes up this capital or lives diminished until death. Qigong can replace this lost energy, enabling people to make up any deficit and recover from the stresses of day-to-day-living. The practice of qigong and neigong each day gives you the energy you need for the day, so you do not spend down your capital or reserves. Likewise, even more practice can add to your reserves.

Your Core Reserve of Energy Is Critical

Obviously, through eating nutritional food, getting appropriate exercise, and living moderately, one can generate a certain amount of life energy that can be used on a day-to-day basis, improving general well-being. Unfortunately, this regimen may not add to the body's core energetic reserves, and one must realize that prolonged stress can burn up these reserves so rapidly that illness may occur. Core reserves are meant for emergencies and disasters, not for daily activity.

The person who lives intelligently will have more than the average energy reserves left to help recover from hard times, but the person who increases core reserves can go from being poor to being rich. This increase in internal wealth, unlike material wealth, cannot be taxed or stolen, and it cannot come from manipulating other people's capital—it must be earned.

When a person's energetic reserves increase significantly, most of the aches and pains, tensions, and general physical discomforts of life vanish. The practice of these core exercises, or tai chi, is a direct investment in the future, just as small daily investments of money when it is compounded can lead to large sums down the road. Herein is not the path of instant gratification, though almost immediately there will be a sense of increased well-being and body ease. The real value of these exercises will become obvious as the years go on, as the energy or capital gained grows even larger.

Qigong's Fundamental Principle: Heaven, Earth and Man

All tai chi chuan practices, as well as those of qigong, are based on the fundamental Chinese concepts of Heaven, Earth and Man *(Tien, Di, Ren)*. Energy from the Earth is drawn upward from the practitioner's root; the root being slightly below the spot where the feet touch the earth. Energy descends from heaven through the crown of the head. We are in the middle, and need to receive energy from both of these sources, which in effect are like positive and negative poles. When the positive and negative are connected, the life current can flow naturally. This current can be used on a day-to-day basis, and with training it can be stored in the body like electricity is stored in a car battery.

The Components of Standing

The energetic foundation of the six core exercises in this book, and which permeates all qigong, is standing. Learning to stand begins with the physical alignments of the body. If the body parts are not properly aligned, energy will leak out or dam up, as water would in a poorly constructed plumbing system. Most of the places where these blockages or leakages are first observable in the human body are in and around the joints.

The Descending Chi Current: From Heaven to Earth

The first stage involves bringing energy from heaven through the body and down to earth, which is purely an energetic process. A fundamental principle of qigong and neigong training, unfamiliar to most people in the West, is that the energy moving from above to below is basically responsible for general well-being.

The energetic system in the human body is a bit like an electrical system. Before power can be put through a wire, the system must have the correct insulation and resistance. If such is not the case, the system can burn out or short-circuit. From the Chinese point of view (or from the Indian yogic viewpoint), it is not all that difficult to develop plenty of energy. The difficulty lies in creating a system strong enough to use this current, rather than be damaged by it. Therefore, much of the beginner's time is spent developing the safety measures and internal resistance necessary to ensure that the system is not damaged by adding too much energy too quickly.

This consideration means that in any qigong or neigong practice, before energy is sent through specific circuits, the body's capacity to withstand the increased current must be developed. The greater the amount of power to be put through an electrical system, the thicker the wires, and the heavier the insulation needed.

In qigong and neigong, the system's capacity is increased by developing the downward current of energy. This clears out blockages and strengthens the ability of the central nervous system to hold energy when the current rises upward. Therefore, in the beginning, a much greater proportion of time and practice is spent on grounding energy than on raising it.

Many people temporarily experience involuntary shaking when standing. This shaking is symptomatic of bound physical or emotional energy releasing from the body. This is the same situation that often occurs when someone is getting an acupuncture treatment, except that the release of bound energy can make the needle vibrate rather than your body. Commonly, when an acupuncture needle is inserted into a blocked acupuncture point, the blocked energy grabs the needle and vibrates it. Once the energy blockage is removed, the needle ceases to vibrate because the acupuncture meridian opens.

As energy blocks are cleared by the downward current, energy that has been blocked in the body for long periods of time is freed up, and the body can use this energy easily and comfortably. The only general symptoms that can be disconcerting here are those that occur after the clearing out of very strong blockages. In such instances, there will be a temporary feeling of strong fatigue, as toxins are released from the body and the body undergoes a transition from a lower to higher energy level. This should not be a source of concern, and it is generally considered a sign of progress. Once this transition is complete, the practitioner will have more energy and vitality than before.

The Ascending Chi Current: From Earth to Heaven

The second phase involves bringing energy up the body, from below the ground to above the head, or from earth to heaven. In many schools of energetics, this is the current that is primarily emphasized because of its spiritualizing effects. This is the phase where people tend to begin having "spiritual experiences," such as psychic experiences, visions, internal sounds, and out of body experiences as well as, to be honest, all manners of hallucinations, spacing out, and general disassociation from the body.

When energy is flowing evenly, powerfully, and naturally through you, you will experience a sense of comfort, ease, and relaxed clarity. It is blockages that create sensations. These experiences can seem to be either positive or negative. What needs to be understood about them is that they are all just essentially experiences of energy blockages. If the blockage feels bad, a person wants to "work through it," and a sense of achievement comes from emptying the garbage.

Experiences of lights, sounds, visions and other psychic phenomena are assumed to be great boons, to be coveted and possessed at all costs. The classic hook used to control people in all sorts of manipulative energy practices involves getting them to think that they are special, or more powerful or elevated than other people simply because they have these paranormal experiences and can project energy in odd or unusual ways. This can easily lead people to substitute these psychic experiences for alcohol, cocaine, and other addictive substances, in effect creating an energy junkie. Although this form of energy work is a much more positive addiction than drugs or other obsessive behaviors, it still is not the true intent of these exercises.

The sense of well-being and clarity that comes when energy is flowing smoothly does not have the incredible power surges and larger-than-life quality to it that many imagine. It is, rather, just a very natural ease and connectedness to oneself, to one's normal interactions in life, and to one's physical, mental, and spiritual bodies. When the shoe truly fits the foot, the shoe is forgotten, and one just walks, easily and comfortably.

Humans Must Balance These Currents

In the Chinese internal energy practices, eight units of time and effort are usually spent in developing the descending current and two units of time and effort in developing the ascending current, so that all the safely precautions are in place before too much juice is put in the system. Many people throughout history, in many countries and traditions, have concentrated almost exclusively on the upward current, and a tremendous amount of unnecessary burnout has been the result. See Appendix C for further information.

The Chinese realize that energy is always around and has always existed, and through the power of the mind its forms can be changed greatly. The mind, through its capacity to project, is able to direct the chi, using the medium of the central nervous system. Chi is bound with blood in the human body, and this chi-infused blood has the ability to reach every cell of the body.

The nerves play a critical role in qigong practice, and are the metaphorical wiring that we discussed before. It is through the transformation of the nerves, the actual physical nerves, that the chi can be effectively and safely directed by the mind. The nerves of the human body take longer to develop than almost any other tissue, and once developed they do not change as rapidly as other tissues. This means that the longer and more steadily qigong is practiced, the more permanent and long lasting the effects will be. Qigong works to permanently change the nervous system with slow, steady practice.

Do Not Skip Steps in Qigong Training

While there is a fair amount of theory included in the material herein, this book primarily teaches the practical application of many principles of qigong and is meant to be used as a workbook. Consequently, the lessons are presented in sequence, step by step, with suggestions about how much time to spend on each. Each piece builds upon the previous one, and you must let an individual lesson stabilize (that is, be able to do it with ease) before you move on to the next. If you jump ahead in your practice, you may, besides wasting your time, find yourself creating a weakness in your energy structure, and it often takes many times as long to correct this kind of weakness as it took to acquire it. Therefore, take your time, and for maximum benefit do not leap ahead in learning these exercises, even out of curiosity, but work with each one as it comes up. If you merely want to satisfy your intellectual curiosity, reading ahead will not matter, but if you want this material to manifest practically in your life, you must actually practice the lessons and the steps within them in sequence.

The human mind is capable of receiving a tremendous amount of information simultaneously. However, there is a world of difference between receiving something and being able to assimilate and use it. Scientific studies indicate that the human mind can only assimilate approximately seven "bits" of information at any given time before it overloads and basically scrambles the information. In qigong, the mind is asked to understand and co-ordinate the material, and the tissue and nerves to remember it.

Qigong requires both intellectual and physical comprehension. The kinesthetic sense of balance, energy, and internal body activities is significantly more difficult to learn than the intellectual information. A Ph.D. cannot assume that his mental capacities will help him to play the game of handball faster than someone of lesser scholastic level. No matter who you are, qigong must be learned slowly and gradually. There is no reason to feel anxious if you progress at a rate that seems slower than that of those around you.

Cultivate Your Chi Slowly, with Frequent Repetition

After more than thirty-five years of teaching these movements to large numbers of people of varying ages, physical capacities and intellectual talents, I have found that the way people learn qigong best is through deliberate repetition. When things were not deliberately repeated over and over again in classes, people stated that they understood, but in fact did not.

So, take your time and follow instructions carefully. I would not say that qigong is easy to learn, but I would say that it is not all that difficult, especially when you consider its incredible benefits.

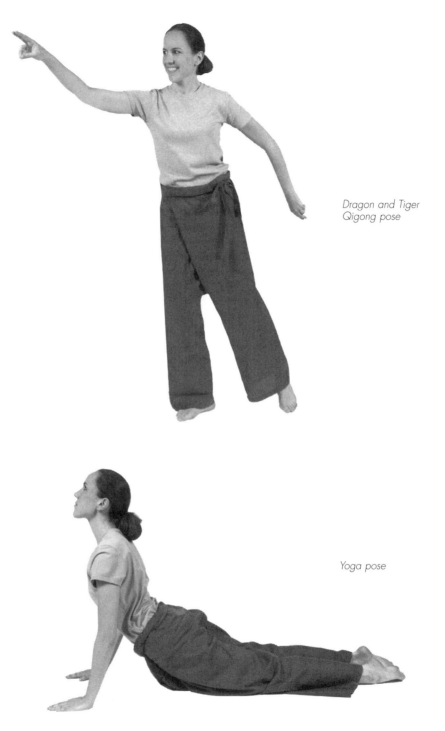

Dragon and Tiger Qigong pose

Yoga pose

Mette Heinz

Health and longevity are goals of both hatha yoga and qigong. Many people cross-train in both disciplines. Both emphasize stretching, breath and energy work.

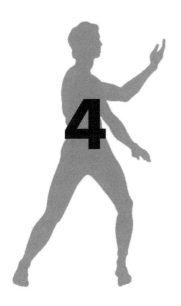

4 Qigong and Other Exercises

All exercises are not the same. Even though they may all be concerned with moving your body, they can result in extremely different physical, mental and emotional experiences. Although both qigong and other exercises are affecting your body and changing you, different parts of you are involved in varying degrees. For example, although running and qigong improve the circulation of blood in the body, they achieve this in quite dissimilar ways (see p. 34 and p. 39).

External Exercise

External exercises usually move your torso and limbs in a forceful, sustained manner. Run, jump, bend, move your arms, lift those legs, work those muscles.

They are primarily aerobic: they stimulate and increase the activities of your heart and lungs, strengthen the large muscles of your body and help keep you in shape. They relieve stress by raising your level of endorphins (natural sedatives) and catecholamines (mood elevators). They may also help relax muscles that have become tense from stress.

External exercises include weight training, bicycle riding, running, rowing, power walking, calisthenics, step dancing, jazzercise, etc. Most Western sports are extensions of external exercises and incorporate them into their training. As exercise, most forms of martial arts, such as karate, tae kwon do and kick boxing are also external in nature.

Internal Exercise

Internal exercise is about training you to feel and change all aspects of your inner ecology: physically, emotionally, energetically, mentally, psychically and spiritually. It is more than just being aware of what is in your mind or training it to be more competitive, aggressive or more highly motivated to accomplish your goals.

Most people have not been trained to feel deeply inside their bodies. Although most people can feel their large muscles move and feel and locate pain, they cannot feel much else.

This is because they have not been trained to know and to feel how their bodies work. For example, if you ask people whether they can feel their liver or their kidneys, many will not even know where these organs are located, much less be able to feel them.

Internal exercises progressively train you to feel the deep physical and energetic states inside your body and how they influence your mind and spirit. As you learn to access deeper levels, you will work with the most subtle and powerful forces within yourself. Internal exercise creates the possibility of enhancing your conscious awareness of the mind and body.

Depending on the exercise system, focus will be placed on some or all of the following—physical alignments (biomechanics), breath, energy and spirituality—to help increase your level of awareness.

Exercises that are primarily internal include Taoist energy arts such as qigong, tai chi and bagua; classic hatha yoga; and Taoist and pranayama breathing.

Some forms of Western exercise, such as Pilates and the Feldenkrais Method, combine external exercise and some aspects of internal training. Increasingly, sports coaches and external martial arts instructors are incorporating internal elements from Eastern and Western systems into their trainings.

Alignments: Biomechanics

At a beginning level, the external aspect of internal training is biomechanics. Biomechanics teaches how different parts of the body can be aligned and trained to move most efficiently. The foundation elements start with the physical alignments of the body (posture) and look at how alignments and movement affect coordination, energy flow, emotions, etc. Biomechanics deals with the following questions:

- How do you correct conditions such as a hunched or stooped back; a collapsed midriff; fallen arches; and tense shoulders and back muscles?

- What is the best way to coordinate the physical movements of your limbs so that they work together in a relaxed, synergistic and whole-body fashion?
- How do different qigong and yoga asanas, body alignments, postures and movements affect your tension and stress?
- How can tension be released, not just from your muscles, but from deeper within your body, such as from ligaments, tendons, joints, tissues, internal organs and bones?
- How can the alignments of your muscles, bones, ligaments and joints progressively be made to work together at higher levels of efficiency?
- How can you originate or power the movement of one part of your body from different or multiple other parts with specific internal muscle or joint sequencings?
- How can you use alignments to control your flow of energy?
- How can your body, mind and energy align to move simultaneously and well?

Although all these questions are connected with biomechanics, the specific methods for answering them differ among various exercise systems. For example, the Western military posture—shoulders and chest thrust back, belly sucked in and tense, joints stiffly held—may help induce the anger and aggression commonly associated with fighting and battle. The qigong posture—relaxed joints, chest rounded, belly relaxed—helps promote balance and calmness of mind. This posture is also a major component of the internal martial arts (tai chi, hsing-i and bagua).

Although training in the most sophisticated biomechanic methods is probably missing from your average gym, it is being increasingly incorporated into sports medicine, professional and Olympic training, as well as in some amateur sports and martial arts.

Breath

Eastern and Western medical practitioners have long recognized the importance of the breath to health and the release of tension. Breath training is part of most internal exercise systems and is also increasingly a part of Western sports training. Breath training is a part of learning to quiet the mind in many meditation and prayer practices.

Chapter 5 talks about differences in Western and Eastern breathing practices and teaches some of the basic techniques of Taoist breathing.

Energy

The flow of chi through the body's energy channels was mapped thousands of years ago. This map is as precise as any electrical wiring diagram. The basis of some Eastern medical systems and their associated exercise systems is concerned with becoming aware of, balancing, unblocking and stimulating this flow of energy through all its channels in the body. For example, a common goal of Ayurvedic and Chinese medicine is to balance the energies within us. However, the methods they use to achieve this within their herbal, acupuncture and medical massage traditions are very different.

Spirituality

Many Eastern physical exercise systems have at their core a spiritual tradition. For example, this book's Taoist qigong is based on the meditation tradition of the Tao as passed down by Lao Tse and the *I Ching*. Hatha yoga is based on the *Yoga Sutras* by Patanjali of which many interpretations and commentaries have been written.

In both yoga and qigong, physically-based internal exercises are preparatory phases of their respective spiritual paths. However, both can be practiced with only the goals of enhancing health, reducing stress and quieting the mind.

Taoist Qigong Is Primarily Internal

The benefits of the core qigong exercises taught in this book are mainly accomplished by working at progressively more sophisticated levels with biomechanics, breath, energy and spirituality. Emphasis is placed on feeling how your movements impact such functions as:

- The expansion and contraction of your tissues.
- The circulation of the fluids in your body.
- The flow of your energy and nerve impulses.
- The pressurization and massaging of your internal organs.

Qigong increases your conscious awareness of your internal body functions and enables you to change and improve them.

Qigong Leads You into Neigong

The most complete version of the Taoist approach to qigong is the 16-part neigong system (see Chapter 15). Here you learn to become aware of and directly affect all your subtle energy flows that power your physical body, emotions and thought patterns.

Neigong helps you deal with the subtleties of how you connect all the disjointed parts of everything that is you, until all your energy patterns become strong, smooth and full in a balanced way without blockages.

You will begin with the physical components of energy just under your skin and progressively move to directly affect and balance the energy in all your muscles, ligaments, joints and spine and finally your fluids, internal organs and glands.

When the awareness of your body and energy is prepared sufficiently, you will learn the more sophisticated internal exercises of meditation that work with the energies of the emotions, psychic realm and most importantly, what those in the East call karma. This level of internal exercise requires not only considerable subtlety and commitment but also the courage to deal with the pain, expectations and negative emotions inside you.

Qigong Improves the Body/Mind Connection

Qigong is an effective, systematic way to improve your coordination, regardless of your age or body type.

Your brain controls your muscles via your nervous system. Some people, especially natural athletes, have marvelously developed nervous systems and they need only be shown a movement to be able to do it. However, such people are a minority of the population. Also, the speed and facility with which the nervous system learns decreases with age for the average human being. A ten-year-old will learn any athletic function much more rapidly than someone forty or fifty.

Fortunately, the ancient Chinese Taoists developed these qigong techniques to train the nervous system to better link the mind and body and help you avoid needless struggle.

Qigong body/mind techniques are especially useful in any endeavor where physical coordination is important—physical exercise, athletics and dance.

Qigong Is a Good Internal Warm-up for Other Exercise Systems

The core exercises of this book are useful as warm-ups for athletics, yoga and dance. They are, however, quite unlike the stretches and other movements that a runner, yoga practitioner or karate fighter performs. The functions of these qigong warm-ups are to:

- Make your mind as quiet and stable as possible.
- Bring all the internal connections between your various body parts and your mind into operation.
- Raise the efficiency of your internal organs.
- Open your spine and your joints to increase flexibility, agility and speed.
- Promote healing and prevent injuries by increasing your awareness of your body's limitations on any given day.

If you practice the core exercises for a long time, you can develop a relaxed power and flexibility that is usually unobtainable to the average person.

The internal martial arts of tai chi, hsing-i and bagua are, for many people, too complex and time-consuming to undertake, and the apparent complexity of their movements lead many to become discouraged and quit. The exercises in this book have the advantage of having very few external motions, which allows you to devote your time and effort purely to internal development. When learned thoroughly and practiced diligently, these core exercises allow you to learn an internal martial art much faster and with less frustration.

Cross-Training with Qigong

It is common for athletes and practitioners of all types of exercise systems to cross-train to enhance performance of the primary activity.

To figure out if you should or should not cross-train, it is logical to base your decisions on some kind of cost/benefit analysis and to talk to your current and potential trainers, teachers and coaches. How much time and money do you need to invest in learning? Which type of training will help the primary activity? What are your goals? Are they to make you faster, stronger or looser? Does one type of exercise create higher physical functionality but not affect your appearance or vice versa? What are the risks associated with the exercise? Here are some of the common trade-offs you may want to consider:

Consciously Tensing or Relaxing Muscles and Joints

Many exercise systems are based on either tensing or relaxing your muscles. For example, weight training requires that you tense muscles, and karate kicks and chops require you to lock your joints and tense muscles at the point of contact; whereas qigong requires that you consciously relax your muscles and other internal parts and never lock your joints.

Tensing muscles can be useful for body sculpting—creating a buff body. Although most qigong improves performance, it does not affect appearance in a dramatic fashion.

You can acquire strength, speed and power with tension; or you can have them with relaxation. Qigong is well known for making people faster and more fluid. By creating internal strength and balance through relaxation, you will gain better speed, usable power, coordination and flexibility. Relaxed, loose muscles move faster than tense ones.

Qigong increases the speed with which chi circulates through your nerves and body fluids. This is important because the impetus for physical speed, reflexes, muscular relaxation and fluidity of movement comes from your nerves: the more relaxed they are, the faster your response time between thought and action, either physically or mentally. The ability to achieve your speed, power and fluidity relies on the smooth movement of all your body's fluids, not only the blood that carries the oxygen, but also the cerebrospinal, synovial and interstitial fluids that directly affect your spine, brain, joints and cells.

Chi circulation makes it easier to link and coordinate all the parts of your body so that they work together smoothly and efficiently. Tension and sluggish chi impede coordination.

Qigong training is unlikely to cause injury and is easy on the joints, which is especially important for older people.

Tradeoffs for Yin and Yang Personalities

In Taoist practices, everyone is considered to be a combination of yin and yang elements. Yin is thought of as having the qualities of water and yang having the qualities of fire. Your nervous system leans either toward being weak or strong, yin or yang, and this determines how you manifest various physical maladies and attitudes toward life.

If you ask Chinese medical doctors about whether you should do a particular type of exercise, they would answer that question in terms of whether you are primarily a yin or yang personality.

Yin is associated with feminine qualities, such as yielding, calmness and softness. But at the extreme, yin qualities can weaken the nervous system and result in physical sluggishness and emotions that are lackadaisical, passive aggressive, depressed or neurotic. The negative health tendencies of primarily yin personalities are towards gradual decreases of function, slowly fading towards death.

Yin personalities naturally gravitate towards, and benefit more from, exercises that are gentle, soften the muscles and release tension. Practicing qigong and tai chi will improve the constitutions of yin people. They generally do not achieve the same results with yang exercise, regardless of how strong their grit and will power. The strain of hard physical exercise is difficult for yin nervous systems to accommodate and yin people will easily quit yang types of exercise.

Although many exercises reduce depression to some degree by getting the body active, the gentleness of qigong can be especially helpful to those who need physical activity that will not strain their weakened nervous systems. Once qigong relaxes and strengthens a weakened yin personality, he or she may find it helpful to add gentle yang exercises, such as light resistance training or walking.

Yang is associated with so-called masculine qualities such as aggression, force and straining to achieve goals. Yang nervous systems are found in type A personalities. Yang personalities are easily prone to anger and physical tension, and they can be adrenaline junkies. The negative health tendencies of primarily yang personalities are likely to consist of sudden deterioration: they go and go and then have a sudden heart attack or stroke.

Yang personalities naturally gravitate toward yang exercises, such as running or weight training, highly aerobic "killer" workouts, or aggressively competitive sports, such as football or basketball.

When doing any cross-training exercise, yang personalities that primarily do yang type exercises should ask these questions:

- Does draining off excess adrenaline cause your energy to feel spent and depleted, even after you have had a short rest?
- Are your nerves more wired or strained?
- Doess the exercise usually release emotional turmoil and increase the tendency to get frustrated and lose patience? If the answers to these questions are yes, it is time to add a yin exercise program like qigong that will help bring relaxation.

Likewise, if yin people have done qigong and tai chi exclusively for years and still answer yes to these questions, they should cross-train with a more yang exercise system, such as light resistance training or Pilates, to add more yang balance to their systems.

Stress-Reducing and Stress-Producing Exercises

Although most Western doctors say that any exercise reduces stress, the perspective of Chinese qigong doctors is different. They would ask what kind of stress you are experiencing and look at how a particular exercise would reduce or exacerbate that stress.

Stress is experienced in your body, emotions and mind. Today's electronic age has produced a sedentary population where many people push their minds and nervous systems dramatically more than they push their muscles. Stress can make you feel nervous, sluggish or in pain. It can be experienced as emotional exhaustion, uncontrolled negative emotions and frequent mood swings. Moreover, stress can drain and diminish your mental energy, focus, clarity and creativity.

If your central issue is body stress, it may be that primarily yang aerobic exercises, such as running, which pump and oxygenate your blood, burn off stress hormones and rouse competitive spirit, will help you combat your stress.

However, if emotional and mental stress are more noticeable, you need to release the physical tension and habitual contractions in your muscles; the built-up tension in your nervous system; and the blockages in your energy channels. In this case, add soft, yin kinds of exercises like qigong and tai chi, which soothe, release, balance and regenerate energy channels and nerves.

Qigong Is Good Cross-Training for Golf and Weight Training

Qigong enhances the performance of many athletes and external martial artists. In this section, two popular sports, golf and weight training, are used as representative examples of high and low impact exercises to provide an understanding of how qigong can be beneficial.

Weight Training

How can qigong, an exercise system based on relaxing and softening muscles, help weight trainers whose goals are to make their muscles hard, strong and shapely?

Qigong reduces the downside of weight training while improving its benefits. It enables you to increase your flexibility, strength and rotational ability. Qigong improves your coordination and brings power from your legs to your arms. Qigong reduces the time that a practitioner needs to regenerate before attempting another repetition.

Weight training can make muscles overly hard and tight, which limits their range of motion. If they move too far in some direction, or if one muscle holds stiff and another pulls on it, the result can be muscle sprains, tears, rotator cuff damage or damaged backs. Qigong decreases the risk of damaged muscles and backs and hyperextended joints. It increases your internal sensitivity and helps you to know when you are overstraining.

Weight training can increase your body tension and trigger adrenaline releases, emotional explosions and anger. Doing qigong reduces your tension and stress triggers, while allowing you to build muscle tone and strength.

Golf

Golf and qigong, which are physically low impact exercises, have many similarities. Both are relatively gentle forms of exercise. Both focus on coordinating hand movements with weight shifting and waist turning to get the parts of the body to work together. Both develop patience and mental focus. Both seek to develop power and better performance through relaxation, speed and precision of movement rather than with muscular tension or brute force. Leaving aside the emotional reactions of frustration and anger that some golfers may experience, golf and qigong, being physically low-impact exercises, have little potential for negative consequences to the body.

The core exercises in this book include three swings (Chapters 11, 12 & 13). These train golfers to turn correctly in either direction and shift their weight without negatively impacting the knees. They provide greater stability on the weighted leg, which results in a better platform from which to launch a swing or make a putt.

The Cloud Hands exercise taught in this book links the body in ways that increase hand sensitivity and power, providing the needed control for long and short putts.

The swings loosen your shoulders, hips and waist to provide relaxed power to drive the ball.

The first swing loosens the rotating abilities of your leg muscles, which are used to turn and shift your weight smoothly as you turn back to power your stroke. The first and second swings allow you to derive power from your legs and back and transmit it through your arms, which is critical for hitting the ball a long way. The third swing uses the same basic up and down arm motions as a golf swing and helps connect your arms and legs so that they move together as you turn and shift your weight.

These swings help loosen all your muscles and joints, which can help you play any sport.

All the core exercises in this book help to balance both sides of the body.

Hatha Yoga and Qigong

Hatha yoga and qigong are the two main approaches from which all non-Western types of exercise are derived.

Hatha yoga uses postures (*asanas*) and breath control (*pranayama*) to energize subtle channels (*nadis*). Qigong uses movement and breath to move and balance chi.

However, the methods and strategies by which they realize their goals are different. In hatha yoga you stretch in order to relax, whereas in qigong you relax in order to stretch.

Hatha yoga asks you to stretch into a posture or asana as much as you are capable of and hold it, often with some amount of tension in your body. You then relax and release the pose. Strong emphasis is placed on will power and control.

With any movement of qigong, you are asked to find the point that is approximately 70 percent of maximum physical extension or range of motion, and when you find it, as much as possible, relax everything in your body, mind and spirit. The goal is to release your nerves, which enables everything in your body to naturally relax and lengthen. Strong emphasis is placed on continuous, conscious relaxation until your body lets go of its tension and naturally stretches.

Qigong Can Improve Hatha Yoga Practice

Qigong's internal training can tune you in to how the different asanas are affecting your deep physical and emotional layers. Qigong's emphasis on softening gives your nerves the ability to release your muscles so that they can have the flexibility you need to get into and hold yoga's postures.

Qigong will increase your awareness of the movements of your chi or prana energy as you do the asanas. Its emphasis on moderation keeps you from overstretching, which can lead to injuries.

Taoist Yoga

For thousands of years, Taoists in China have had their own version of yoga. Instead of using movement like qigong, it focuses on assuming and holding postures that are similar to hatha yoga postures.

Taoist Qigong	Hatha Yoga
Most qigong is primarily done standing upright and while continuously moving.	Postures held in static, unmoving positions and most are done on the floor.
No extreme positions at any level of practice.	Intermediate and advanced levels do extreme stretched positions.
Theory, fundamental approach and practices based entirely on circularity.	Linear in theory and approach, limited amount of circular movements.
Medical perspective based on traditional acupuncture and Chinese medicine.	Medical perspective based on India's traditional medicine, Ayurveda.
Energy work based on chi and principles of acupuncture and developed through the internal techniques of the Taoist 16-part neigong system.	Energy work based on prana, mantras and chakras and developed through visualization, energy and breath exercises.
Emphasizes 70 percent rule, never locks joints or extends range of motion to 100 percent.	Normally emphasizes going to 100 percent extension.
No back bends or inverted positions.	Many back bends and inverted postures.
Advocates never tensing any muscle in the body. Accomplishes relaxation through continuously releasing all tension in the nerves and muscles.	Advocates tensing a muscle so it can relax afterwards.
Breath never held.	Breath often held.

Taoist yoga poses are primarily done on the floor and are similar to simple hatha yoga postures. Taoist yoga shies away from difficult stretches, such as that of putting your feet behind your head. A soft approach is emphasized. Taoist yoga focuses on working with nerves and energy channels.

The system that the author has developed to teach Taoist yoga is called Longevity Breathing® Yoga. You begin with a very minimal stretch. Then, using Taoist breathing techniques and following the principle of never deliberately tensing your body, you increase the stretch by relaxing and deliberately unblocking the energy inside you. The goal is to learn and progressively incorporate all the principles of Taoist neigong within each posture (see Chapter 15). This includes releasing blocked energy within acupuncture points and channels; pulsing the fluids in your joints, internal organs and spinal vertebrae; and manipulating the energy within your etheric field or aura.

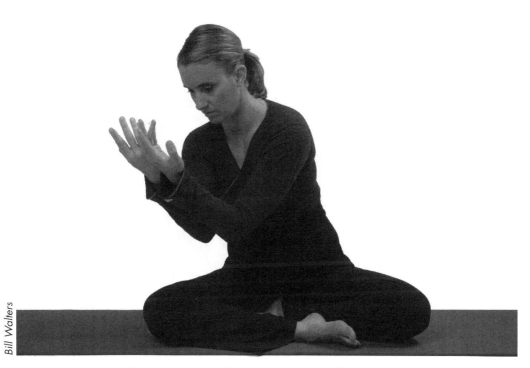

Bill Walters

A basic Longevity Breathing Yoga pose derived from Taoist yoga.

Richard Marks

The author teaches Longevity Breathing, helping a student to relax her diaphragm and breathe into her belly.

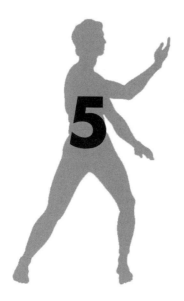

5   Breath and Chi

Both Western and Eastern medical practitioners consider good breathing habits to be exceedingly important components of health, relaxation, longevity and spirituality. Although most people are aware of when they eat or sleep poorly, relatively few pay attention to or notice how they breathe.

Unfortunately, many people breathe poorly—they take shallow breaths without fully engaging their lungs. As people age, they experience shortness of breath, which is a precursor to ill health, weakness and depression.

Of all self-help exercises, learning to breathe properly is one of the most effective ways to improve your overall health and at the very least, mitigate the decline of aging. That is why Taoist energy practices start with breathing.

This chapter will teach you the basics of the Longevity Breathing program, the foundation for Taoist qigong and other energy and meditation practices. The techniques are easy to learn, although practice is required.

Taoist Breathing/Longevity Breathing: What's the Difference?

Taoist breathing is fundamental to all Taoist longevity practices. Although these practices are thousands of years old, I have developed my own method for teaching them, namely the Longevity Breathing program. As a Taoist lineage holder, I must ensure that Taoist practices are taught accurately and represent the tradition. Longevity Breathing makes these practices accessible and easy to learn, particularly for Westerners. These methods may be quite different from those that other teachers use to teach Taoist breathing.

Breathing with Your Belly

Longevity Breathing begins with breathing from the belly. It is patterned after the way babies breathe. Everything inside a baby's body moves in rhythm with the breaths. As the baby's lungs fill with air, all the internal organs, tissues and blood vessels expand. Babies have incredibly strong breathing mechanisms. They can cry or scream for hours and move around constantly to a degree that would exhaust most adults.

Think of your belly as a cylinder and your breath as a means to expand that cylinder equally in all directions from its centerline. In the direct center of your body, about two to three inches below your navel, there is an important energy point that the Chinese call the lower *tantien* (called the *hara* in Japanese). Your belly goes from your lower tantien up to your solar plexus (the first soft spot you hit when you tap down from the middle of your breastbone) at your diaphragm muscle and back to where the diaphragm meets your spine (see p. 84). Your belly area includes your liver, spleen, stomach and kidneys; it does not include your chest or ribs.

Although having a flat, contracted belly may make you look fit and attractive, it does not make your body relaxed and can lead to health problems as you get older. Keeping your belly tight and compact is usually only accomplished and mantained through habitual tension, which can shorten the ligaments that are attached to your internal organs, as well as compress the internal organs and cut off blood flow to them. Tension held in your belly for a long time can lead to ulcers, hernias, digestive problems, etc. Many people experience negative emotions and anxiety directly in their bellies.

The goal of Taoist breathing is to relax your belly so that it can expand and contract with your breathing. This fully engages your diaphragm, brings air to all parts of your lungs, improves blood circulation to your internal organs and relaxes your nervous system.

What Longevity Breathing Accomplishes

The basic nature of Taoist breathing is to get everything inside your body moving in synch to the rhythm of your breathing. It makes the inside of your body fully alive, joyful and healthy. It cultivates your ability to relax at any time and concentrate on what you are doing for long periods without becoming distracted. Longevity Breathing accomplishes these goals by:

- Facilitating the abundance of oxygen and the balance of oxygen and carbon dioxide in your body.
- Ensuring that carbon dioxide is fully expelled.
- Retraining your nervous system to relax.
- Improving the functioning of your internal organs.
- Increasing the levels of chi in your body.

Increases Oxygen Levels

The oxygen in your blood powers your metabolism, circulation and your ability to heal. Decreasing levels of oxygen makes you prone to illness, morbid emotions and weak physical and mental performance.

Most Western doctors recommend aerobic exercise as the best way to increase the volume of oxygen in your body.

Longevity Breathing methods will do the same. When qigong is practiced along with Longevity Breathing, the flow of oxygen will become smooth and balanced throughout your body.

Gets Rid of Carbon Dioxide

Longevity breathing gets rid of carbon dioxide and increases the usable oxygen that you inhale.

Even if you can inhale sufficiently to pull enough oxygen in to your system, you might not exhale deeply or long enough to get rid of all the carbon dioxide required. Normally a quarter or so reserve at the bottom of the lungs is always filled with carbon dioxide. This leaves only three quarters of the lungs free to be filled with oxygen, or remained unused. As the exhale relative to the inhale becomes even weaker, it diminishes the ability of the body to procure oxygen from the air.

If you do not exhale sufficiently, over time, these events may occur:

- The ability of your body to procure oxygen from the air diminishes.
- Toxic waste products build up in your blood, which often results in yawning.
- As carbon dioxide builds up, your mental capacities and clarity diminish and your stress level increases.
- Increased carbon dioxide accumulation beyond what is naturally needed prevents your lungs from taking in enough air.

Helps You Relax

Longevity Breathing helps you create and stabilize a strong, steady breathing pattern that will mitigate excessive emotional swings. It retrains your nervous system to relax and make your thoughts smoother and more comfortable.

Studying your breathing patterns can make you aware of the ways you move into your moods and emotions. For example, fear tends to produce erratic, strained or weak breathing patterns. Holding your breath is often a precursor to violent, angry explosions. Likewise, holding your breath without realizing it is part of a reaction to stress and tends to increase its severity. Shallow breathing makes people prone to lung weaknesses in the face of environmental problems, such as polluted air, and can lead to depression.

Improves the Functioning of the Internal Organs

According to traditional Chinese medicine, the ability of your breathing to improve the functioning of your internal organs—liver, kidneys, heart, etc.—is as valuable as increased oxygen. Longevity Breathing emphasizes using the pressure that your breath can generate within and around your internal organs to massage and drive more blood and chi into them and optimize their natural range of movement.

If this range of motion diminishes, blood flow to your internal organs will also diminish. This will block the smooth flow of energy. Other effects include the gradual shortening of your ligaments and restricted movement of your organs. Bodily functions will gradually weaken and disease will eventually strike.

Taoist qigong, and other Eastern breathing practices such as pranayama, teach specific breathing patterns that can induce specific emotions in the practitioner. Some Taoist schools combine breathing with such meditation techniques as inner dissolving to transform the negative emotions within your energy channels to balanced and positive ones, such as generosity and compassion.

Longevity Breathing Practices Are Fundamental to Taoist Meditation

Within the Taoist tradition, qigong and meditation form a continuum. Qigong can lead you to meditation. Breathing can help you to feel the inside your body and the deepest recesses of your spirit and soul. It gives you access to your emotions so that you can move towards realizing your greatest potential by releasing everything that is bound inside you.

Longevity Breathing is a tool to awaken your awareness so that you can see into the center of your soul. As breathing energizes your body, it enables you to recognize how the chi of your emotions and karma is frozen. You can then dissolve and release what is stuck inside until the blocked energies resume their natural free-flowing quality and you can begin to walk the path called the Tao.

Taoist Breathing and Pranayama Yoga

Eastern medicine has brought two major breathing systems to the West: one is pranayama or yogic breathing; the other is Taoist breathing. Taoist breathing and pranayama breathing practices have many similarities:

- Both use breathing techniques to teach you to make conscious contact with your own chi or prana.
- Both seek to extend the duration of your inhales and exhales.
- Both advocate good posture while breathing, although with some differing views as to what good posture is.
- Both advocate breathing techniques as a way to age well and reap the benefits of longevity.
- Both advocate breathing techniques as a way to create physical, mental and psychic power.

However, they also have some fundamental differences. Many core practices of pranayama breathing teach you to hold your breath or to breathe in or out of one nostril.

In Longevity Breathing, your breath is never held: your goal is relaxed, circular, whole-body breathing. This means that Longevity Breathing can be done 24 hours a day, once the technique is mastered.

Most pranayama methods focus on breathing from your chest. Taoist methods focus on breathing from your belly.

Taoist Qigong	Pranayama Yoga
Does not breathe into the front of the chest.	Breathes into the front of the chest.
Can be done 24 hours a day.	Cannot be done 24 hours a day.
Never holds the breath.	Sometimes holds the breath after inhale or exhale.
Strong emphasis on kidney breathing.	Lesser emphasis.
Diaphragm developed by expanding downward and causing increased pressure through the internal organs to the lower belly and tantien.	Diaphragm developed by rapidly lifting and dropping it through such techniques as the bellows breath or the lifting contraction of the abdominal muscle to massage the digestive system (*uddiyana bandha*).
Breath always done with both nostrils.	Uses alternate nostril breathing where one nostril is closed while the other is open.

Learning Longevity Breathing

Longevity Breathing is learned in systematic stages. Breathing is the first component of Taoist neigong, with methods from the simple to the complex (See Chapter 15).

In the beginning stage, you train your breathing so that eventually every internal part of your body is consistently and powerfully engaged. This requires effort and regular practice.

This phase involves learning to breathe into your belly and abdomen and bring breath all the way up the back of your lungs. Besides taking air in and out of your lungs, different parts inside your body must expand and contract in coordination with each inhale and exhale. The parts of your abdominal region that must be engaged with every breath are the diaphragm, and the front, sides and back of your belly, including your lower back and kidney area. You will also learn not to inhale air into the front of your chest.

This is the only stage of breathing taught in this book. If you continue your study of qigong, you will learn more complex methods, some of which are discussed in Chapter 15.

Breathing Benchmarks

The Longevity Breathing program has three benchmarks based on the duration of your breath. The first is thirty seconds (fifteen-second inhales; fifteen-second exhales). This is the only benchmark that beginners should try to reach when they learn the Longevity Breathing techniques taught in this book. A thirty-second breath is the minimum an average person should be able to achieve in order to breathe well under normal circumstances. Being able to do this easily is quite a challenge, but achieving it will immeasurably better your life.

The second benchmark for more advanced practitioners is a two-minute breath, and the third is five minutes or longer. These are discussed more fully in Chapter 15. Under no circumstances should the breath ever be held.

If, after taking four or five deep breaths, the longest you can extend an individual breath is ten seconds (five-second inhales; five-second exhales), your normal resting breath is likely to be three to five seconds and even less under stress.

Anatomy of Longevity Breathing

Your diaphragm moves air in and out of your lungs. It is a bell-shaped sheet of muscle that separates your lungs from your entire abdomen (Figure 5-1). It wraps around the lower parts of your rib cage and attaches to your spine. Your diaphragm moves when you breathe. The bell shape flattens and your chest cavity and lungs expand and draw in air. When your diaphragm relaxes and resumes its bell shape, your chest gets smaller and causes air to be pushed out of your lungs. If your diaphragm does not move very much as you breathe, you cannot take in or expel much air.

Your diaphragm influences a complex variety of interconnected anatomical parts—upwards to your head, neck and shoulders and downwards towards the bottom of your pelvis—to move in coordination with it.

Spongy, springy ligaments connect your diaphragm to your internal organs and cause them to move in coordination with your breathing. For example, if your diaphragm moves well, it makes your liver move well. If the movements of your diaphragm are poor, it can cause the ligaments that connect to your liver to lose function. A poorly functioning liver will compromise your other internal organs.

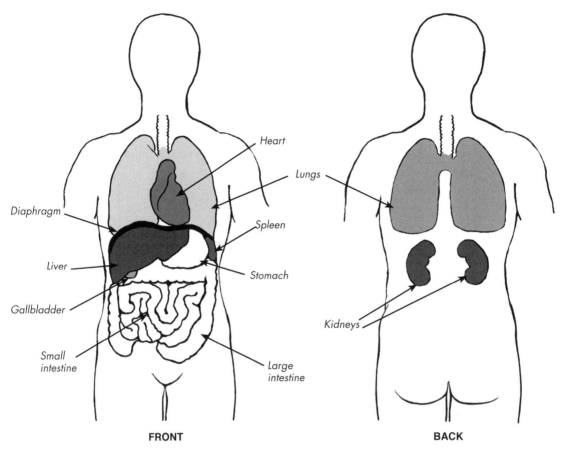

Heart

Lungs

Diaphragm

Spleen

Liver

Stomach

Gallbladder

Small
intestine

Large
intestine

Kidneys

FRONT

BACK

The Internal Organs of the Body
Figure 5-1

Your body has several internal fluid pumping mechanisms, which are directly connected to the movement of your diaphragm. Good fluid movements are especially important for your internal organs, joints and spine. Poor movement of your diaphragm compromises the smooth flow of these fluids.

The Longevity Breathing exercises that follow will help your diaphragm to move more strongly and teach you to develop habits of long, strong and deep breathing.

Guidelines for Learning

As you do the Longevity Breathing lessons below, adhere to these five guidelines:

1. Breathe Softly in a Relaxed Manner

Just as muscles can tense up and become hard, so can your breathing. Breathing powerfully but softly and in a relaxed manner can reduce the tendency of your nervous system to become stressed or hold onto stress. Soft breathing, rather than tense or labored breathing, enables you to shrug off stress and negative emotions significantly more easily.

2. Breathe Through Your Nose

Longevity Breathing is quiet breathing. The goals are to fill your lungs, calm your nerves and get your chi to flow strongly. The best way all these goals can be met is to breathe through your nose. However, if you have medical problems and have difficulty breathing through your nose, breathe with your mouth slightly open.

3. Remember the 70 Percent Rule

Straining your breathing will involuntarily induce tension. Forcing your breathing can negatively pattern your nervous system and lock in tension. Only breathe to approximately 70 percent of your capacity—in terms of both how long you make your inhales and exhales, and how much you physically move the spaces within your abdomen and lungs.

4. Keep Your Tongue on the Roof of Your Mouth

As you breathe, you should keep your tongue on the roof of your mouth in as relaxed a fashion as you can. (When you start to say "let" your tongue will naturally go to the correct position.) Your tongue may feel tight at first but in a few weeks your muscles will loosen and you will be able to keep your tongue on the roof of your mouth at all times. This contact connects two major energetic flows in your body.

5. Do Not Hold Your Breath

Each breath should flow into the next in a relaxed manner. Gradually decrease the delay between your inhale and exhales so that your breathing becomes smooth, even and continuous.

6. Do Not Breathe into the Genitals

In this form of breathing, you should not feel any physical pressure anywhere below the area of your pubic hair (See Appendix C). Other Taoist techniques for breathing into the genitals are specific to Taoist sexual practices.

How Long Will It Take to Learn Longevity Breathing?

This is a common question and the best answer is, "As long as it takes." Letting go of your internal sense of time pressure to succeed can help you accomplish this task in as short a period as your body and nerves will allow.

Classically, Taoists considered that a minimum of three months (or one of the four seasons) of regular, almost daily practice was necessary to enable new breathing patterns to become as natural as all other physical activities and occur even during sleep. The very disciplined may be able to achieve this in less time, while the less disciplined may need a year or more. To put it simply, just practice regularly and forget about how long the process should take.

Practicing with discipline at regular times for regular amounts of time is ideal. However if this is not possible, practice whenever you can, such as while watching television, riding on a bus, plane or train, waiting for appointments or emails to arrive, doing household chores, etc. If you miss a time to practice breathing, don't feel guilty. Just take the next opportunity. Over time, small steps can travel great distances.

Lesson 1 Move Your Belly Forward

The position for most easily learning these exercises is lying on your back. Your legs can be stretched out or you can raise your knees, whichever makes you feel the most comfortable. You can also sit in a chair, as long as you gently lift and straighten your spine and do not allow it to slump. (Instructions for sitting correctly are found in Chapter 6.)

Once you can do the breathing exercises sitting or lying down, you can try them standing up or you can incorporate them into your standing, moving, lying down or sitting qigong practice. Your goal is to develop the unconscious habit of good breathing in all circumstances you may find yourself.

1. Review the guidelines for breathing on the previous page.

2. Take a baseline measurement of the duration of your breath. Using the second hand of a clock or watch, breathe comfortably and measure your current rates of inhale and exhale. Do not try to force the length of your breath.

3. Put one hand on your belly and one hand on your chest. Push your belly out to draw in air. To exhale, relax and allow your belly to return to its original position.

4. The front of your chest should stay still and relaxed, neither moving up or down. Let all your inhales and exhales come directly from the movement of your belly.

5. Try to make each inhale and exhale approximately the same length.

6. Start by doing this exercise 5 times during each practice session and increase to 20 as it becomes comfortable. You can practice any time and you will be ready to go to the next exercise when you are comfortable doing 20 belly breaths.

Lesson 2 Bring Movement to All Parts of Your Belly

In the beginning, you may notice that some parts of your belly move more easily than other parts. Commonly, the lower belly moves the most easily and the middle of the belly the next most easily. The part of the belly located just under the center of the diaphragm and the solar plexus is usually the hardest to move.

It takes most people some weeks and sometimes months to be able to feel a distinct and definite movement in their upper belly and solar plexus. This is because those muscles have not been trained to move with breathing and often are tense and contracted.

The best way to learn to engage all parts of your belly evenly is first to focus on the part (lower, middle or upper belly) that moves the most easily and get it to move smoothly and completely without any tightness or constriction; then systematically proceed to focus on the others.

1. Place your hands on and focus on the part of your belly that moves the most completely. Get it to move fully and smoothly as you apply the instructions for the first lesson.

2. Put one hand on another part of your belly. Focus on getting it to move as you inhale and exhale.

3. Do this 5 times during each practice session and increase it to 20 as it becomes comfortable. As soon as this part of your belly can move equally smoothly you will be ready to go on to moving the third part of your belly when you simultaneously move the two other parts strongly for 20 breaths.

4. Focus on the third part of your belly and get it to move just as smoothly.

5. Always remember the 70 percent rule—you should feel as little strain as you can anytime you pratice breathing.

6. Do this exercise 5 times during each practice session and increase it to 20 as it becomes comfortable. You will be ready to go to Lesson Three when you can feel all parts of your belly move smoothly for 20 breaths.

Special Note about Breathing Lessons 3–9

It may take weeks or more to do any of the following exercises in a relaxed manner. Take the time and do not skip ahead. As you practice, you may notice that you will also be able to take slightly longer breaths.

Lesson 3 Move the Sides of Your Belly

Focus on expanding and relaxing the sides of your belly. Side breathing begins from just above your hipbones, moves through the next fleshy bit called your midriff and continues underneath the bottom of your ribs. Train your awareness so that you can focus on this area of your body.

1. Place the palm of your hands or lightly closed fists on the midriff area between your hipbones and your lowest ribs. When you inhale, this area expands; when you exhale it returns to its original position. The hands help you to confirm when you are actually moving the sides of your belly.

2. Move the sides of your belly as you breathe until you can feel some pressure on your liver and spleen, located underneath your ribs (see p. 84).

3. Make sure the front of your chest is not moving as you breathe.

4. Time your inhales and the exhales so that they are approximately the same length. If you are able to take longer breaths without strain, do so.

5. Do this exercise 5 times during each practice session and increase it to 20 as it becomes comfortable.

6. When over time, this exercise becomes comfortable, shift your focus a little. Use each inhale to increase your awareness of tension in your muscles and nerves. As you exhale, do your best to consciously release these tensions and allow your

body to relax and soften. As you become more successful, you will get an increased feeling of space—both within the breath itself and within your abdomen—as well as a greater sense of unobstructed flow within your abdominal cavity, where previously you may only have felt hard, tense and bound muscle.

Lesson 4 Breathe Into Your Lower Back and Kidneys

Breathing into your kidneys (see p. 84) is a very important Longevity Breathing practice. In traditional Chinese medicine, the kidneys are held to be the source of a human's overall vitality, life force and sexual procreative capacity.

Energizing your kidneys through your breath is important in terms of developing a healthy body and a clear mind. Chronic fatigue reflects weakness in your kidneys and fear is held there.

Breathing into your kidneys is harder than breathing into the front and sides of your belly. Initially, it helps to lie on the floor, knees up, soles of your feet on the floor, with the lower part of your back firmly pressing the floor. The pressure of your body against the floor on your inhale and the release of the pressure on your exhale will make it easier to feel inside your body.

1. As you inhale, expand the inside of your body backward from the center of your belly to your spine, lower back muscles and up to your kidneys. You should feel your skin pressing more strongly against the floor. Return to your original position as you exhale.

2. Make sure your chest does not move up and down. Continue to breathe into the front and sides of your belly but focus on breathing into your back.

3. As you breathe, try to feel your kidneys. The kidneys are particularly delicate and easily strained. You should be especially gentle and practice only to within 40 percent or 50 percent of your capacity, gradually building to 70 percent.

4. Become aware of your emotions. Does breathing into your kidneys make you more aware? Does it make you fearful? What are you afraid of? What does that fear feel like? Mentally relax that fear. Tell yourself that what you are doing now,

whatever fear you have, is not going to happen while you practice your breathing. Release your fear-induced tension and as you let go and release that tension, release the emotion.

5. Do this exercise 5 times during each practice session and increase it to 20 as it becomes comfortable.

Lesson 5 Move Your Belly in All Directions Simultaneously

Your goal in this exercise is to make your entire belly come alive. The exercise is best learned while sitting.

1   From the centerline of your body, expand your belly in all directions to inhale. Relax to your original position to exhale. All the parts of your belly—front, sides and back—should expand outwards or move inwards simultaneously.

2. Focus your awareness on any part that does not move properly and practice until it does.

3. Make sure your chest is not moving as you move your belly.

4. Do this exercise 5 times during each practice session and increase it to 20 as it becomes comfortable. You should do this exercise for as many weeks or months as it takes to feel all parts of your belly moving in a relaxed manner in all directions simultaneously.

Lesson 6 Breathe Into Your Upper Back

In the previous exercises, you have focused on breathing with your belly. If you have been diligent in your practice, you will have expanded the breathing capacity of your lungs. In this exercise, you will combine kidney and full belly breathing with upper back breathing.

Your lungs are constructed like bags. If, when you inflate a bag, you hold the back of it still, the bag will inflate forward. This is how most people breathe. Their chests expand.

However, if you hold the front of the bag still, the bag will inflate backwards. This is what you do with the chest in Longevity Breathing. The front of your chest, sternum and chest muscles completely relax and do not move at all as your lungs expand backwards towards your spine.

Combining abdominal breathing with breathing into the back of your lungs fully massages your heart, something that does not occur while breathing with the front of your chest. When you learn this exercise, two forces simultaneously converge to give your heart a continuous massage with each breath. First, greater movement in the back of your lungs allows them to apply pressure to the back, top and sides of your heart, which abdominal breathing alone cannot fully accomplish. Second, the upward pressure applied by your abdomen and diaphragm creates a wave of pressure in the bottom, side and front of your heart. These two forces compress and release the entire heart muscle and pericardium in a toning, rhythmic massage.

Having a heart massage is good for you. Since in Chinese medicine, your heart governs anxiousness and anxiety, if you focus on relaxing it while you breathe, you may find your anxiety lessening. As you inhale, bring a sense of gentle confidence into your heart. As you exhale, release your tension, fear and worries about the future.

Breathing into your upper back, combined with belly breathing, also massages, tones and increases the blood circulation of other internal organs.

Most people have never breathed with their upper backs and the tissue of the back part of your lungs is probably not very flexible. As you learn this exercise, remember the 70 percent rule. Take it easy. Do not try to do too much too fast. Gradually, your lungs will regain the stretch they had when you were a baby.

1. Lie on your back with your knees up, the soles of your feet on the floor and the lower part of your back firmly pressing the floor. Put your hands on your chest to check that it does not move.

2. Expand your belly to inhale, but put your focus on letting the muscles of your upper back move backwards. The front of your chest (the sternum and chest muscles) should relax completely and not move at all, as your lungs expand backward towards your spine.

3. As you inhale, relax your shoulders. Allow your shoulder blades to spread away from your spine as you let your ribs and shoulders soften and move sideways. This action will release some of the anatomical bindings that prevent your lungs from fully expanding.

4. As you exhale, try to feel the back of your lungs releasing air, the muscles of your upper back relaxing and your shoulder blades moving closer towards your spine.

5. Do this exercise 5 times during each practice session and increase it to 20 as it becomes comfortable. Do this exercise until you can feel all parts of your belly moving in a relaxed manner in all directions simultaneously as the back of your lungs fill.

Breathe this way many times during the day until you make breathing from your belly and upper back something that you do all the time without having to think about it, regardless of whether you are standing, moving, sitting, lying down or talking.

Important Points to Remember

The more you practice Longevity Breathing, the more it will improve your health and relaxation. Be patient with yourself. Poor breathing habits will fall away as you practice.

Eventually, you will have clear sensations that each breath is massaging your internal organs and spine. Your breathing should be consciously developed until it can cause everything inside your body to move in direct coordination with each inhale and exhale.

Take the time to notice how each breath has a distinct quality of feeling. Once you recognize this, you can, by conscious intent alone, direct this feeling to any area of your body. This is an invaluable aid to gain control of your body, consciously work with your emotions and directly feel chi.

Consciously directing your breath is a powerful tool for gaining the ability to recognize how your blood and other fluids are moving inside you. Over time, it is important to gain the ability to use your conscious intent as you breathe to get fluids to move evenly and strongly inside your body.

1. Your Diaphragm Will Stretch Very Slowly

Take your time and make sure you stay well within your comfort zone when your increased breathing capacity begins to stretch areas inside your body, including you diaphragm. Stay well within your 70 percent capacity. You may find that small sections of different parts of your diaphragm are tighter or looser than others. When attempting to loosen a tighter part, just breathe into it until it stretches a bit more. If you have a loose part, then breathing into it will help it develop more tone. Your goal is to make your diaphragm evenly stretched and springy.

2. If You Are Injured, Do Not Overstrain

Keep in mind that the strength of any bodily movement when you are injured is keyed by your breathing. In this sense, breath is a double-edged sword. More breath gives better oxygen, which can help an injury heal faster. Conversely, it may cause you to unconsciously move the injured area excessively and thereby retraumatize it and slow your healing process.

3. Remember the 70 Percent Rule

As your breathing gets more powerful it can make you aware of pain. Any clear or dramatic escalation of pain is a sign that you are not adhering to the 70 percent rule.

4. Keep Your Emotions Steady

If you find that focusing on increasing your breathing increases negative emotions, such as anger or fear, back off and shorten the duration of each breath. Make sure your emotions smooth out before you refocus on increasing the duration.

5. Do Not Be in a Hurry

Organic, self-sustaining growth takes time. Beware of sabotaging your progress by being in too much of a rush.

Breathing and All Qigong Movements

As you learn the six core exercises that follow or any Taoist qigong movement—standing, moving, sitting or lying down—as best as you can, maintain a relaxed, even and steady breath. Do not hold your breath. The tendency for many is to have their breath get weaker and weaker until they start involuntarily holding it without knowing they are doing it. Use the Taoist breathing techniques in this chapter to maintain a strong and vibrant breath as you exercise and, most importantly, in your daily life.

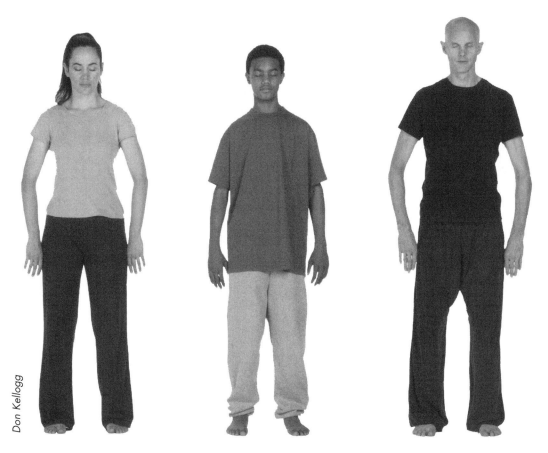

Don Kellogg

Standing and dissolving energy blockages is a core practice of Opening the Energy Gates of Your Body Qigong. This powerful technique increases internal awareness and develops more chi inside your body.

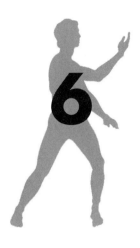

6 Basic Standing and Sitting Alignments

Six Core Exercises

The core exercises in this book are composed of six elements: the first is the fundamental neigong standing posture, taught in three parts: sinking, scanning and dissolving your chi.

The second is Cloud Hands, which integrates the internal principles learned in the standing postures into moving your body as one coordinated synergistic whole. Here, you also learn some of the coordination basics common to tai chi and other Taoist qigong energy practices, such as turning your torso and coordinating your arms and legs.

The third, fourth and fifth elements are swing movements, which open the joints of your arms and legs and infuse your internal organs with energy.

The sixth element is a spinal stretch, which has the primary function of gaining control of your vertebrae and their related nerves and chi flow.

Body Alignments

The body alignments incorporated within the standing and sitting postures for the core qigong exercises taught in this book are fundamental to all Taoist energy practices. These are the basic physical alignments that allow your body to relax. They enable fluids and chi to flow in a smooth, balanced manner. They teach you how to stand and sit properly.

Tension that has locked into various parts of your body contributes to poor posture and may cause physical discomfort, such as back and neck pain.

Practicing these exercises will gradually enable you to move your body into correct alignments, relax your tension, become healthier and free your energy. Take the time to learn and practice each lesson thoroughly before going on to the next.

Although standing is recommended, these exercises can be done sitting in a chair. Thus, people that are ill, bedridden, wheelchair bound or otherwise too weak to stand can do them sitting. The exercises can also be done by alternating between standing and sitting. Instructions for the sitting postures will be found later in this chapter.

Lesson 1 Standing Alignments

The standing posture called *Jan Juang* or "stand strong" is a powerful meditation used to develop internal power *(Figure 6.1)*. Some qigong masters use this method alone as their daily practice. It is fundamental to qigong, neigong, and tai chi chuan, as it opens the energy gates of the body and thus allows the free movement of chi. In the next three chapters, the techniques of standing are described in a series of sequential lessons. The material in each lesson must be practiced and understood before moving on to the next. Both body and energy mechanics are discussed in each lesson.

Placement of the Feet

Your Stance Must Be Comfortable

Begin standing with the outer edges of your feet somewhere between hip- and shoulder-width apart, wherever you find it to be most stable and comfortable. The appropriate stance will become more obvious with practice and depends on the relationship between the width of the hips and shoulders. A person with wide shoulders and narrow hips will generally want a stance closer to hip width, while a person with narrow shoulders and wide hips will tend towards a stance closer to shoulder width.

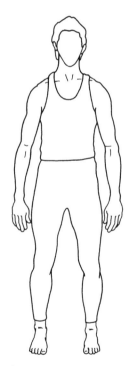

Standing posture. Feet are parallel, shoulder-width apart.

Figure 6-1

Eventually, the center of each foot should align with the left and right energy channels of the body.

Keep Your Feet Parallel to Each Other

The knees should be slightly bent and the feet parallel. Parallel placement of the feet means that the distance between the toes is the same as the distance between the heels, and one foot is neither in front of nor behind the other *(Figure 6-2)*. For example, if the feet are fifteen inches apart, then there should be fifteen inches between the big toes of each foot and fifteen inches between the heels of each foot and each knee.

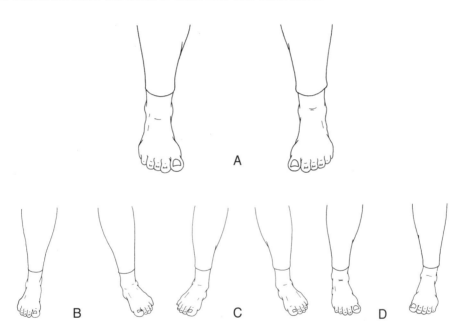

A) Correct: Feet parallel. B) Incorrect: One foot splayed outward.
C) Incorrect: Both feet splayed outward. D) Incorrect: Feet turned inward.
Figure 6-2

Placement of the Spine

Your Tailbone Should Point to the Ground

Your tailbone should be perpendicular to the floor *(Figure 6-3)*; it should not incline backward, as it does when you stand normally. The lower back, from the tailbone up to and including the lumbar vertebrae, should be relatively straight. In most people, the spine naturally has an "S" shape, with curves at the bottom, middle, and top. In the standing posture discussed here, however, the lower part of the spine is straightened.

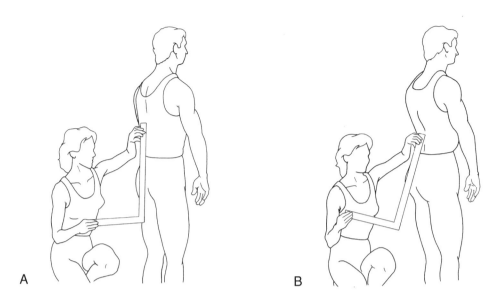

A) Correct: Lower back straight, perpendicular to the floor.
B) Incorrect: Lower back curved, buttocks protruding.

Figure 6-3

Gently Straighten Your Spine

Your spine should be straightened by 1) gently rolling your hips under, and 2) using your inner back muscles to push the kidneys slightly back. Together, these two processes will make the lower part of your spine totally straight.

Obviously, human beings come in various and sundry sizes. For those of thin or medium build, the easiest way to determine if the back is straight is to check if the buttocks are protruding backwards. If this is the case, the posture is not correct. For those of heavier build, the buttock may give the impression that the back is swayed even when the back is in fact straight. For this type of physique, the important point is that the back and sacrum are straight, and not whether the buttocks stick out.

The rest of the back should be kept fairly straight and should not lean in any direction.

Placement of the Neck and Head

Your Head Should Float Lightly Above Your Neck

The neck and head need to be held straight *(Figure 6-4)*; the crown of the head is straight up so that a line drawn straight up from the crown would be perpendicular to the ground.

As the neck and shoulders relax, quite commonly the head will want to tilt. It is preferable that the head remain upright, but although a slight forward tilt is acceptable *(Figure 6-4B)*, any backward tilt is not *(Figure 6-4D)*. Also, it is important to gently lift the occiput from the atlas vertebra (that is, lift the skull gently off the neck bone) to reduce compression of the neck vertebrae. The Chinese liken this to the feeling of lifting a hat off a coat rack.

This essential element of qigong, which will hold true for all movements of the core exercises, is called *ding*, or raising the head. *Ding* stretches the spinal cord of the neck area, making sure that the weight of the skull 1) does not compress or misalign the vertebrae of the neck and 2) does not close down the flow of chi and/or nerve energy from the hind brain to the spinal cord. Such closure occurs if pressure is brought to bear on the atlas/axis, the last vertebra at the base of the skull. This principle of *ding* must be present during all standing, moving or sitting qigong practices. To do this, first hold the neck completely vertical. The jaw is then drawn slightly back, so the eyes and jaw are exactly parallel to the ground and the crown of the skull moves vertically upwards. This action stretches the vertebrae of the neck and lifts the skull slightly. It must not be done in such a way as to create any tension or stiffness in the jaw, neck, head or shoulders.

The Eyes and the Tongue

Beginners Practice with Eyes Shut; Tongue Touches Roof of Mouth

In standing, your eyes should be kept initially closed to facilitate your going inward. There are many practices where the eyes remain open, but these are not recommended for beginners. Beginners usually need all their concentration

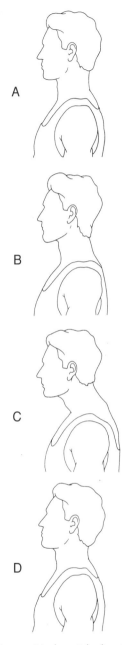

A

B

C

D

A) Correct: Neck straight, head lifted. B) Incorrect: Head slightly forward. C) Incorrect: Head forward, chin out.
D) Incorrect: Head back, chin out.

Figure 6-4

to keep track of what is occurring internally, without attending to the external environment.

The tongue should be kept touching the roof of the mouth during all qigong practices, with the tip of the tongue against the roof of the mouth behind the front teeth. This action is necessary in order to complete the microcosmic circulation of energy in the body. The point of the roof of the mouth is where the major yang and yin energies of the body meet. If you say "let" the tip of the tongue will naturally arrive at the correct spot.

Placement of the Chest

Gently Allow Your Chest to Sink as It Rounds

Han shiung ba bei, or "round the chest and raise the spine" is a fundamental technique found in all Taoist meditation, internal martial arts, and qigong practices, regardless of school. *Han shiung* means to have a half chest, or a chest shaped like an hour glass: that is, it is rounded on both the vertical and horizontal planes. This is like the posture of a baby, where the chest is very relaxed, the shoulders are relaxed downward, and the belly is rounded, dropped and relaxed *(Figure 6-5A).* The standard Western military pose, with the chest thrown out, stomach in, and shoulders and buttocks pushed back, is the exact opposite of this *(Figure 6-5B).*

Your Chest Should Expand Toward Your Navel and the Sides of Your Ribs

It is very important to understand that in no way should you collapse or depress the chest. This will simply cause the diaphragm or lungs to be compressed. In dropping the chest, it remains relaxed so that, from the inside edge of the shoulders (below the end of the collarbone—what the Chinese call the shoulder's nest) all the way through the belly to the hips, there is a sense of sinking, dropping, and opening downwards. At the sides, there is a sense of the chest and ribs softening and spreading, allowing the chest to attain its full size without being compressed.

This is based on the principle that the tantien, the area in the lower abdomen where chi is stored, is like a reservoir or bowl, and that by relaxing the chest downwards, the chi will drop from the upper body and collect in the lower tantien. If the chest is raised up, the chi will rise upwards rather that sink, which commonly will result in an angry or overly forceful or aggressive disposition. In the external martial arts this is called *ti shiung,* which means "raising the chest." *Ti shiung* creates the classic V-shaped body, with overdeveloped chest and arm muscles.

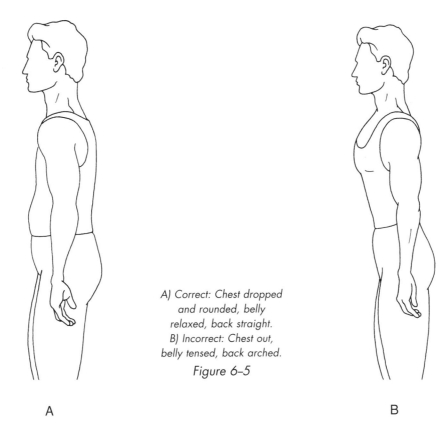

A) Correct: Chest dropped
and rounded, belly
relaxed, back straight.
B) Incorrect: Chest out,
belly tensed, back arched.

Figure 6–5

A   B

Your Chest Should Stay as Soft as a Baby's

Han shiung (the rounded chest) is based on the fundamental Taoist proposition that one should make one's body like that of a child, as children are totally natural, unconditioned beings, and as such are wonderfully and naturally efficient. Children, especially babies before they have begun to imitate their elders, have big bellies and relaxed chests. For their size, babies are stronger and more filled with energy than adults. Try to feel the strength a child has for its size, and how relaxed it is. Also, note how babies can scream for hours without any trouble. Most adults cannot keep up with a baby.

The Taoists found that children and animals (also not conditioned) have something in common. Both breathe from the belly and have a relaxed chest, so that the internal organs drops downward and are massaged by each breath and movement of the body. Observe cats or dogs, cows or horses, and see how their bellies swing from side to side as they walk. This "squishing" of the internal organs strengthens them, in much the same way that massage makes the muscles of the body healthier and stronger.

Give Your Organs an Internal Massage

Gladiators in ancient Rome were massaged every day during training and especially in the mornings before a contest so that they might give a good show. The same effect can be brought about through this relaxing of the chest and dropping of the internal organs. In the classic V-shaped body, the internal organs are pulled up, placing them in fairly fixed positions, which segment the body into upper, middle, and lower thirds. This reduces internal pressure and causes internal organs to receive much less massage through breathing and movement than if the chest were relaxed and dropped.

Internal pressure is extremely important, in that it causes the endocrine system and the glands of the body to maximize their secretions. A similar internal pressure is created in hatha yoga (which also develops the classic "V" shaped body). In hatha yoga, however, rather than all the endocrine glands of the system being affected simultaneously, specific exercises exist for each gland. In standing postures and neigong work in general, all systems are worked simultaneously. The end result of this relaxation of the chest is to allow energy to drop to the tantien, where it is stored like money in a great body bank account, to be used as necessary.

Raise Your Spine and Spread Your Shoulder Blades

Ba bei refers to the raising of the spine. The lungs need to expand and open in order to breathe. In the V-shape body practices, the chest is pushed forward (convex), and the back arched as the shoulder blades rise up and converge towards the spine. Conversely, the raising of the spine (back) in neigong causes two things to occur.

First, the spine physically rises up, as if it were being pulled upwards. This takes some of the curve out of the upper back. The term *ba* in Chinese means to pluck something up, like pulling grass or a plant out of the ground. So as the chest is moving downwards, the back and spine are raising upwards, which allows the lungs plenty of room on a vertical plane.

Second, on the horizontal plane, the back becomes totally rounded *(Figure 6-6A)*. Instead of the shoulder blades coming together as they do in the military posture *(Figure 6-6B)*, they relax downward, spread as far apart as possible, so that the lungs expand backwards towards the spine. When these two principles are combined with the straightening of the lower back, the net result is a series of yin/yang balances that are the opposite of the standard military V-shaped posture.

In the standard military posture, the chest is out, and the rear end has shifted backwards. In the Taoist position, the chest is rounded into a half moon shape, and the back is flat with the pelvis tilting forward. In the military posture, the stomach is sucked in and the chest raised up, while in the Taoist posture the chest is relaxed downwards and the belly is dropped. In the military posture, the bottom and top of the spine are clearly curved. In the Taoist posture, they are basically straight.

The Taoist posture also makes it easier to breathe naturally from the diaphragm, in the way that opera singers and babies do. Taoist consider this way of breathing to be ideal for adults.

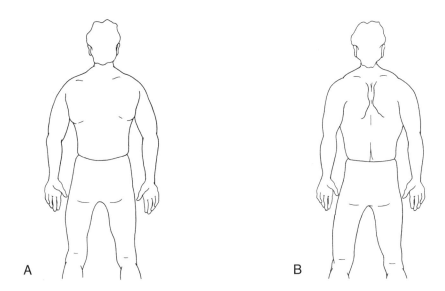

A) Correct: Shoulder blades spread, shoulders rounded forward.
B) Incorrect: Shoulder blades drawn toward spine, shoulders pushed back.

Figure 6-6

Small Heavenly Orbit: Internal Organs Sink as Spine Rises

From the pelvis up to the ribs, on the sides of the body (at the midriff), the internal oblique muscles should perform a lifting or raising action to prevent downward compression, which allows the vertebrae of the lower spine to remain straight, with plenty of intervertebral space. This muscular lifting is done simultaneously with the front of the body sinking downwards, so that in the trunk of the body, between the solar plexus and the hips, there is a sinking as well as a rising.

The lifting of the spine and the dropping of the internal organs and chi together create the Small Heavenly Orbit of Energy, sometimes called the Microcosmic Orbit or Small Circulation. This is called *shao jio tien* in Chinese, and has been openly written about and practiced for thousands of years in China.

There are deeper, more secretive and esoteric aspects of this practice, however, that must be learned under the strict guidance of a teacher to prevent bodily harm. The material in this book regarding the circulation of energy is fairly common knowledge in China among people who do this kind of work, and is quite safe to practice. Some energy practices are kept secret because to reveal them to a general audience would be like putting a gun in the hand of a child. Many things are not taught in qigong until a certain amount of experience and maturity is established in the student.

Palms Face Backwards as Hands Rest on Sides of Thighs

This posture is the most energetically neutral pose. It is ideal for beginners practicing standing. This position specifically keeps the armpits open so that the left and right energy channels (see p. 238) do not close down. For beginners, the thumbs lightly touch the sides of the thighs. Let the space between the thumb and index finger, called the Tiger's Mouth in Chinese, relax and naturally spread.

Lesson 2 Sitting Alignments

The Taoist sitting posture described below emphasizes achieving relaxation through breathing from your belly and the back of your lungs.

Other recommended techniques to alleviate physical tension and pain for people that sit for prolonged periods of time, such as office and computer workers, and people who practice sitting qigong and meditation, are described in Appendix D.

Basic Sitting Posture

The chair you use should be one with a flat, unmoving bottom with at least an inch of free space on each side of your hips and a solid, unmoving, straight back set perpendicularly to the seat. The seat should be of a height so you can sit, with your feet flat on the floor with your knees bent at an angle of approximately 90 degrees *(Figure 6-7)*. The alignments of the sitting posture mimic in all major respects the alignments of the standing posture.

- Keep your spine straight *(Figure 6-7B)*. To straighten your spine initially (or later on

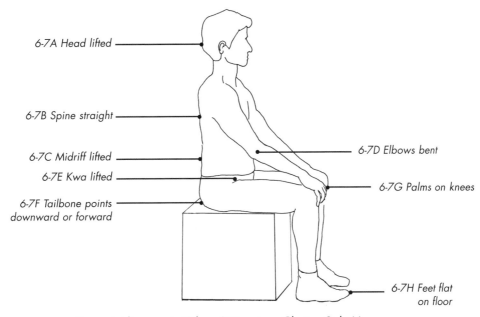

6-7A Head lifted

6-7B Spine straight

6-7C Midriff lifted

6-7E Kwa lifted

6-7F Tailbone points downward or forward

6-7D Elbows bent

6-7G Palms on knees

6-7H Feet flat on floor

Correct Alignments When Sitting in a Chair—Side View
Figure 6-7

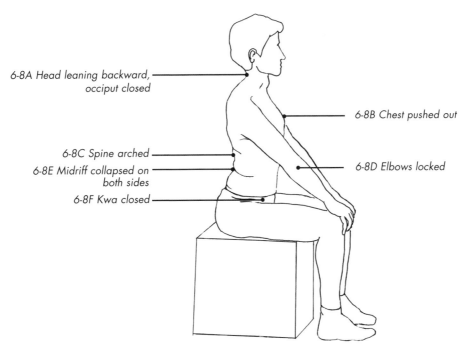

6-8A Head leaning backward, occiput closed

6-8B Chest pushed out

6-8C Spine arched

6-8E Midriff collapsed on both sides

6-8F Kwa closed

6-8D Elbows locked

Incorrect Alignments When Sitting in a Chair—Side View
Figure 6-8

if it begins to sag during practice), lift upwards from the front of the spine. The more you can relax the front of your throat, chest, and belly, the easier this lifting will be. If you tire and feel the need to bend your spine forward, focus your mind on relaxing the back part of your spine. (The methods for learning to control the separate movements of the front and back of the spine are taught in the Advanced Spine Warm-up 1 section of Chapter 14.)

- Your midriff *(Figure 6-7C)*—the space between the top of your pelvis and the bottom of the ribs and kwa *(Figure 6-12A)* are gently straightened upwards to create more physical space within the top and bottom of each. In most people, these habitually collapse and slump during prolonged sitting, to the detriment of the spine. The area of the body that the Chinese call the kwa extends from the inguinal ligament through the inside of the pelvis to the top (crest) of the hip bones (see p. 163).

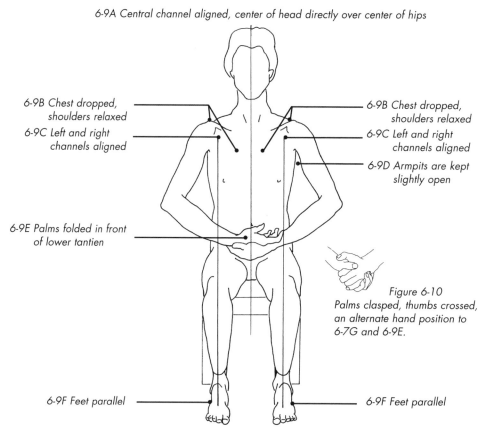

6-9A *Central channel aligned, center of head directly over center of hips*

6-9B *Chest dropped, shoulders relaxed*

6-9C *Left and right channels aligned*

6-9B *Chest dropped, shoulders relaxed*

6-9C *Left and right channels aligned*

6-9D *Armpits are kept slightly open*

6-9E *Palms folded in front of lower tantien*

Figure 6-10 Palms clasped, thumbs crossed, an alternate hand position to 6-7G and 6-9E.

6-9F *Feet parallel*

6-9F *Feet parallel*

Correct Alignments When Sitting in a Chair—Front View
Figure 6-9

- Your armpits should be kept open, elbows slightly bent and your arms held slightly away from your torso *(Figures 6-7D and 6-9D)*.
- Your chest and shoulders should be relaxed *(Figure 6-9B)*.
- Your head should be lifted gently from the top of the neck *(see Figure 6-4A, p. 99)* and positioned directly over the center of the torso and pelvis *(Figure 6-9A)*.
- Your left and right channels should be aligned with the corresponding shoulder's nest and kwa *(Figure 6-9C)*. (The shoulder's nest is the hollow created between the inner edge of the shoulder and the ribs.)
- Your central channel is aligned so that the crown of your head and the center of your pelvis are on a line perpendicular to the floor *(Figure. 6-9A)*.

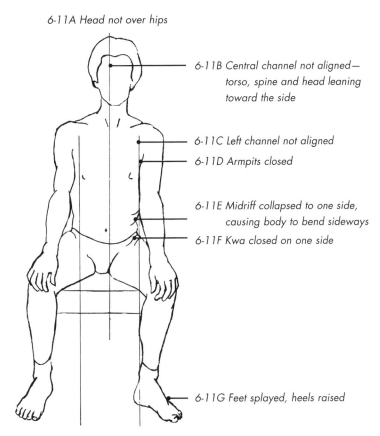

6-11A Head not over hips

6-11B Central channel not aligned— torso, spine and head leaning toward the side

6-11C Left channel not aligned

6-11D Armpits closed

6-11E Midriff collapsed to one side, causing body to bend sideways

6-11F Kwa closed on one side

6-11G Feet splayed, heels raised

Incorrect Alignments When Sitting in a Chair—Front View
Figure 6-11

Lift Your Kwa While You Sit

Figures 6-12A and B show how your pelvis stretches upward when your kwa opens and collapses when your kwa closes. Open your kwa when you begin to sit, and make a special point of checking it at regular intervals.

To open your kwa, lift everything you can feel, from your perineum through your pelvis to the tops of your hipbones, through your midriff to the bottom of your ribs, but without also lifting your chest. When you accomplish this opening maneuver, your inguinal fold will straighten, relieving any discomfort and fatigue you might be feeling.

Your kwa must be lifted gently. Also, do not deliberately contract your anus as is done in some fire method qigong techniques. The anus will be lifted effortlessly by the movement of your kwa.

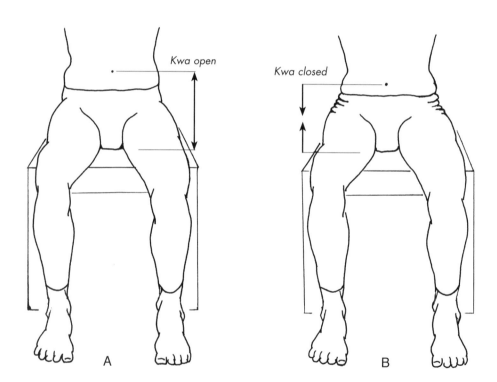

Lifting the Kwa
A) Correct: Kwa open and lifted. B) Incorrect: Kwa closed down.
Figure 6-12

Exercises to Stretch Your Kwa

The exercises described here will help teach you to stretch your kwa while sitting. Gently, press your feet continuously against the floor throughout each exercise to obtain a solid connection from your feet to your spine. Press until your knees feel stable.

When doing any sitting qigong exercise, your hands should remain in one of the positions shown in Figures 6-7G, 6-9E and 6-10.

1. Extend and elongate your muscles from your knees to your lowest ribs

> If done well, this stretching will noticeably release the muscles of your back, shoulders and neck.

2. Bend forward from the kwa. Bend forward from your inguinal fold and return to your starting position

> Keep your torso and head upright as you let your body incline forward then return to its original position. A kwa bend originates its movement of the torso from the kwa and not your back muscles, head or neck. Move slowly and rhythmically so that you gradually stretch your kwa and midriff. This bend will be in the range of from 6 to 18 inches.
>
> • Use the 70 percent rule to know how far to stretch. Bend only as far as you can to comfortably maintain your internal work and relieve your body of any distracting discomfort.
>
> • Remember to keep your spine straight.

3. Stretch your kwa and midriff by moving your body in a circle

> First, lean slightly forward, then to the right, then slightly back, then to the left and then forward again, using the center of your pelvis as the center of your circle. As you execute this circling, it is important to continuously extend and stretch your body from an imaginary line within your body that extends from your legs to your perineum through the center of your body up the front of your spine and out from the top of your head *(Figure 6-9A)*. Pay particular attention to stretching from your knees through your kwa and midriff when you get to the left and right sides of the circle *(Figure 6-9C)*. Do your best to even out any imbalance by moving more

slowly or extending the imaginary line higher on the more contracted side. Pay extra attention to lifting your kwa when moving to the sides.

4. Do between 1 and 3 repetitions, moving both clockwise and counter-clockwise

Lesson 3 Stand and Settle In

Before you can really work with the exercises described in this book, you need to settle down and be fully present, so that you are focused on feeling your body.

As you stand, focus on your breath. Put your tongue on the roof of your mouth and feel your breath as you inhale and exhale. Make it smooth, relaxed and balanced, with no gaps between each exhale and inhale. Do this until you can easily focus on your breathing. Next, breathe into any part of your body that feels numb or tense until it relaxes. After a few minutes, you should find that relaxation is easier and you are more easily able to focus on what is happening inside your body.

Turn your attention to your alignments. While standing, start with the top of your head and work down to your feet. Use your mind to gently go through the alignments mentioned earlier in this chapter. As you focus on the major alignments, feel whether they are in or out and use your best effort to adjust your body position until they feel more correct and stable.

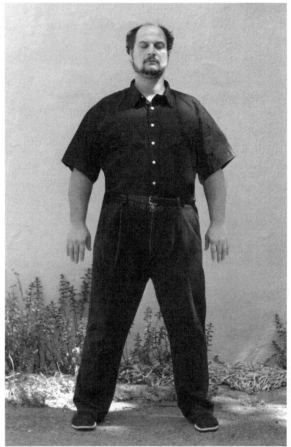

Hideki Matsuoka

The ideal neutral posture with which to begin standing qigong. There are other postures that produce more specific effects.

Breathing into an alignment that is out makes this easier and more effective.

Remember the 70 percent rule and don't attempt to force an alignment into its proper position. If you do not rush, your body will slowly realign itself, particularly as you learn the fundamental standing techniques, which use these alignments (Chapter 7). The realignment process will continue throughout your learning of qigong and other Taoist energy practices andgradually all the alignments will become more comfortable and stable.

This settling in process can take as long as ten minutes, until you become more experienced. With practice, settling in will rarely take more than a few minutes, unless you are starting with a very high stress level.

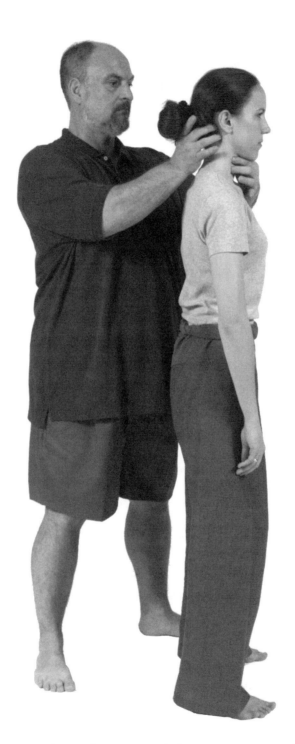

Mette Heinz

Bruce Frantzis adjusts a student's alignments to help improve posture, balance and the circulation of fluids and energy throughout the body.

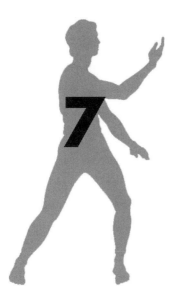

Fundamental Standing Techniques:

Sinking, Scanning and Dissolving Your Chi

Once you have become comfortable with the Longevity Breathing techniques and can settle in to the basic body alignments, you are ready to begin feeling deep inside your body. This chapter teaches the fundamental standing techniques that will help you awaken and feel your chi. There are three lessons: sinking your chi; scanning your energy body; and dissolving chi blockages.

Feeling and working with chi is an art. Remember, the depth, ease and speed your mind can connect to and feel rarified sensations in your body grows over time. The ability to feel your chi will come with that increased awareness.

What Is Sinking Chi?

The first step is to feel any physical sensations of discomfort and tension in your body. These sensations come from places where your chi is blocked and cannot move. Sinking your chi is about feeling these sensations and letting them go. This grounds your body and mind and calms your nervous system. When your chi is no longer blocked, it can make you feel relaxed and full of joy and vitality.

The opposite of sinking the chi is chi rising, the physical signs of which you may experience when feeling anxious. The feeling wells up from your stomach or shoulders and moves towards your head. Your muscles tense. Your breathing may become tense and short or you might hold your breath.

In China, qigong and tai chi masters use the word *sung* when they want their students to feel the physical sensations of tension and discomfort in their bodies and release them by sinking their chi. *Sung* means a complete release, a complete letting go of any sense of control, contraction, strength or binding inside your tissues and nerves, until holding of any kind is replaced by a complete sense of openness, space and comfort.

How the Author Learned to *Sung*

When I first started trying to grasp the term *sung*, I did not have an easy time. In my early days of training in Taiwan, a very friendly Chinese man who was not my main teacher helped me gain the sense of what *sung* meant. I knew minimal Chinese, he was the same with English, and our communications resorted to quite a bit of mime.

My body was tense. He looked up the word *sung* in his dictionary and saw that it was translated as relax. He said in broken English, "You relax no good enough," while mimicking how tensely I was trying to relax my body. I could not let go. Frustrated, he said, "Need *sung*. Have not enough *sung*." He proceeded to demonstrate it to me. Using vastly exaggerated motions, he let his joints go completely loose and stood before me with an obvious lack of any kind of physical tension.

I did not get it. He then demonstrated what he meant with two piles of coins. He put the first pile in a paper bag and laid a knife next to it. He said, "You want *sung* be like money. Make body be like money." Then he took the knife and cut the bag. The coins poured out (letting go of physical tension), fell (releasing the chi downward), separated (loosening the insides of the body), scattered over the floor and soon stopped moving (the body fully *sung*).

I tried again. He saw that I was just half getting it. So he made fists and raised his hands above his navel and suddenly, with his entire body loosening, opened his hands and let them fall to his sides. He grabbed the second pile of coins and brought them up to the same place above his navel and suddenly let go of them. They fell, separated and scattered on the floor. Then just as suddenly, he again let his body relax as his hands and arms visibly loosened and dropped to his sides just as the coins had to the floor.

I put the two images together in my head and got it.

Next, my new friend asked me to touch his arm and belly. He stood with his hands at his side. After checking that I was focusing, he relaxed and without moving an inch, released his body and went *sung*. I could feel his muscles turning to butter and a distinct wave moving down inside his body.

Two-Person Exercise for Letting Go

Many people cannot let go. They are afraid of losing control. This exercise gives you feedback about your willingness to let go.

Person One: Stand with your feet parallel and your hands at your sides. Close your eyes.

Person Two: Lift one of the person's hands to about shoulder height and then lightly and quickly take your hand away so that the hand can fall. The goal is for person one to simply let their hand fall without controlling it. Do this until person one can just let go. Switch roles.

Lesson 1 Sink Your Chi

To feel chi directly you must become open and sensitive to subtlety. Practice each of these lessons in order and only progress to the next one when you are sure that you have absorbed the preceding one.

1. Feel Physical Sensations Inside Your Body

Sinking your chi is a concrete and unambiguously felt internal release. It begins from wherever your mind focuses inside your body, travels downward and finishes either in your lower tantien, the bottom of your feet or in the earth. The feeling of letting go physically should be eventually accompanied by a definite physical feeling of a downward wave inside your body.

First stand with your feet parallel, shoulder-width apart, hands by your sides, palms facing backwards and armpits open. Take the the time to settle your mind and body. The first step is to take a trip through your body from the top of your head to the bottom of your feet, feeling any physical sensations of strength, tension or contraction inside your body. Start by noticing sensations at the top of your head. Then, let your mind slowly travel downward inside your body. Notice where you have any physical feelings of strength or tension. You might feel that the front of your head is tight or that you are tensing your jaw. Your neck and shoulder muscles might feel tense. Do not dwell too long on any one block. Remember the 70 percent rule and do not strain. Feel free to make more than one pass from top to bottom in any practice session—sometimes two shorter passes are better than one that is too slow. Wear down your blocks like water wears rock—a little at a time.

In terms of working with chi, feelings of strength indicate blockages, places in your body where chi is not circulating in a healthy, steady flow. The paradox is this: the more you feel strength, the weaker your chi.

You might also feel sensations of general uneasiness or a sense of contraction inside a body part. For example, when your mind has traveled down to your stomach, you might have angry thoughts come up and you might simultaneously feel your belly contracting.

Uncomfortable physical sensations are reliable indicators of where energy blockages hide in your body. Do your best to feel these sensations, even if they make you uncomfortable. This is common when people first start noticing how the insides of their bodies feel. You may also feel that the sensations intensify when you focus on those feelings.

Travel downwards with your mind, cataloguing these sensations until you reach the bottom of your feet. Start with a minimum of five minutes to go from top to bottom and gradually increase to fifteen minutes or more.

If you cannot stand for this amount of time, you can alternate between standing and sitting. If you do so, place a chair directly behind you to make it easy for you to sit when you need to. Try to transition between your sitting and standing positions very smoothly.

If you are ill or injured, you can do this step seated, until it becomes possible to alternate between sitting and standing and eventually stand for the entire process.

It may take you weeks or months simply to get the experience of recognizing blocked sensations of strength, tension and contraction and to steady your mind enough so it can travel from the top of your head to your feet without becoming distracted. When you can, you are ready to learn to make your chi go *sung*.

2. Sink Blockages Downward and Make Your Chi Go *Sung*

Beginning from the top of your head and moving downwards, settle on whatever physical sensation of blockage your awareness finds first. Then, use your intention in any creative way that works for you to release and let the blockage sink downward or go *sung*.

You will know you have done it when you feel some tangible sensation of letting go and dropping down happening in your body. You might also feel your chi directly, as it moves in a downward wave.

A common error when working with energy is to think you are feeling when in fact you are only visualizing. The feeling of *sung* must translate to tangible and clearly felt physical sensations.

Physical Signs of Sinking Your Chi

Here are some physical signs that will help you confirm if you are actually sinking your chi *(sung)*:

Breathing Relaxes

Although they are not the same, chi and breath are closely related. As your awareness moves down your body or settles on a specific spot of discomfort, your breathing may mirror it. It can suddenly become louder; you may involuntarily hold your breath and it may begin to spasm or flutter rapidly. When you release that blockage, your breathing will become softer, deeper and smoother.

When you find a spot you want to release, you can use your breathing to help. Focusing on quieting your breathing can help release your blockages and deepen your level of *sung*. Letting go of tension in your breathing enables you to release layers of physical tension and helps your chi to sink.

Connect your mind to your breathing while you sink your chi to help prepare you for feeling your chi directly. It will lead you to deeper physical and mental relaxation, soften your body and enable you to increase your awareness of what you feel inside.

Eventually your breathing will become completely silent and you will become able to recognize and consciously work with chi itself.

Alignments Adjust More Easily

The process of realigning your body into the correct standing posture happens slowly. Any body alignment that feels stiff, physically uncomfortable and hard to maintain indicates a place where your chi is blocked.

Sinking your chi through a physical alignment enables you to more easily adjust the alignment and clear the blocked chi. The feeling of blocked chi can intensify when you focus on it. When you relax and let that place go *(sung)*, the alignment will be easier to adjust and maintain.

Muscles Soften; Joints Expand

Hard, stiff, tight muscles will become softer but with significantly more tone. They will move more easily as you sink your chi and release your blockages. The space inside your joints may open, sometimes accompanied by cracking sounds. These can be quite loud, especially in your hip sockets or vertebrae. Normally, this should not be a cause for alarm.

Feet Open

As your chi sinks sufficiently to reach your feet, they can become hot and feel as though they are burning. This is because:

- Small blood vessels within them are open to a greater degree.
- Your metatarsals are getting more space between them.
- Blocked energy in your feet is being cleared.

The Inside of Your Body Increasingly Becomes Wet

The clearest sign that sinking is happening is feeling that either a part or the entire inside of your body is getting wet as your internal fluids circulate more efficiently. The Chinese term for this is *yun chi*.

Chi moves all the fluids of your body. Qigong causes those fluids to circulate more strongly, even through your tiniest blood vessels.

An abundance of chi will make your body feel wet inside, whereas a shortage will make it feel dry. When your body goes *sung* and releases internal tension, you might get a furry or soft feeling inside you, comparable to what you feel after you have taken a hot bath.

According to the *Yellow Emperor's Classic of Medicine*, the fundamental text of Chinese internal medicine, the bodies of young, healthy and vibrant plants, animals and humans are moist and springy. When they move closer to death, their bodies become dry and brittle. People also feel more dried out when they have been ill, tense or after not getting enough sleep. The feeling of dryness occurs when blood and other fluids are not circulating strongly.

When your blood is circulating strongly, the inside of your body feels wetter. As your ability to sink chi gets stronger, it is common for saliva to increase in your mouth. If this occurs, swallow it to reabsorb your chi.

Feeling the inside of your body get wet as you *sung* will give you concrete feedback. This will tell you that you are on the right track. Having a concrete physical sensation, even if it is only fleeting, will help you avoid frustration and not being sure if you are doing *sung* correctly.

When you first start to sink your chi, you are likely to feel the wetness more strongly in particular parts of your body. Eventually, this feeling will spread evenly throughout your entire body. The sensation of your body becoming wet usually begins in your surface muscles and then progresses deeper, until you can feel it all the way to your bones.

As you assimilate the technique of sinking chi, when one specific location in the body gets wet it can increase the sense of wetness throughout your entire body, or one area of your body may cause only another specific one to get wet.

Usually, your body will feel hot just before the sense of wetness becomes obvious. This is a sign of increased blood circulation. It indicates that chi is entering an area and moving through what has been blocked.

As each new release happens, it exponentially increases your ability to release more.

Dropping Your Body and Sinking Your Chi Can Be Confused

When first learning, many feel they must physically move parts of their bodies to act out the internal feeling of sinking, such as bending their knees or lowering their hips. You should strive for an internal feeling of sinking and learn to sink your chi without moving your body.

After sinking has become easier for you, you can combine it with the other core exercises that require moving your body downwards to simultaneously use physical leverage and the power of your chi sinking.

Important Points to Remember

1. As a safety precaution, it is important to first learn to sink your energy flow before engaging in dissolving your chi because that prepares you to handle upward and other energetic flows without injuring your central nervous system.

2. If you are trying to release a particular blockage and you become aware of another one higher up, do not switch your focus to it. Instead, use the following option. Continue sinking from the lower blockage down to your feet and try to ignore the higher blockage. One or both blockages may or may not release of their own accord. If they do not, the blockages may release when you do another downward pass.

3. Adhere to the 70 percent rule.

4. Maintain correct alignments and do not slouch. You should not feel pain inside your joints. If you do, recheck your alignments and if it persists, back off.

Next Level of Sinking

It takes most people months before they can sink their chi to their feet. Begin at the top of your head and systematically try to resolve each individual blockage on the way down. Once you can do this regularly, you are ready to go to the next level and try other specific ways of applying *sung*.

- You can localize *sung* to a specific area without having to first release what is above it. For example, you may notice some tension in your shoulders without needing to begin at the top of your head, and release it by focusing on it and making it go *sung*.
- You can *sung* your entire body and feel a constantly regenerating downward wave of continuous release. Over time, this wave will get stronger and will release deeper and deeper blockages.

Lesson 2 Scan Your Energy Body

Shifting from the Physical to Chi

By this time you should be experienced in sinking your chi. You should have some intermittent inkling now of the possibility that chi can be as tangible as physical sensation. Now you can focus on feeling the sensations of chi itself.

Slowly Observe Any Energy Imbalances in Your Body

Sinking your chi initially only requires you to engage with purely physical sensations. These help you gain awareness of the indirect signs that chi is moving inside your body. Once you have gained that awareness, it is time to directly scan your energy body. This will train you to become more sensitive to your chi and is the preparatory step to dissolving energy blockages.

Beginning at the top of your head, slowly observe any energy imbalances as you scan down your body. These will manifest as places where you feel tension, strength, contraction or something that does not feel quite right. These are the feelings that reliably allow you to locate blocked chi.

1. Strength

Feeling sensations of physical strength are common. Energetic strength is just as tangible, once you become sensitive to feeling the inside of your body. However, what that strength is specifically attached to may be vague. It might be that you have an excess of chi in an area that may also be related to stubbornness or pride. If it feels like blocked energetic strength to you, it probably is. Do not try to analyze it any further than that. Trust your feeling and intuition.

2. Tension

This relates to any two forces inside you that are in conflict, such as physical spasm or where some emotional or mental conflict subliminally lives inside your body.

3. Contraction

The blockage of chi can cause physical constriction in your muscles, internal organs and blood vessels; or emotional constrictions, such as the suppression of anger or sadness.

4. Anything That Does Not Feel Quite Right

These are energetic blockages, which are difficult to verbalize in the mind but are nevertheless tangible, such as general, nonspecific feelings of unease, discomfort, vague pain or places you cannot feel at all. When something feels right you can definitely feel a sense of aliveness in that spot.

Explore your energy body internally, millimeter by millimeter, from the top of your head to the bottom of your feet. Take notice of what you feel. Notice the areas, no matter how small or subtle, that have any qualities of tension, strength or contraction.

Now, pay special attention to those places where you do not know just what it is that does not feel quite right.

It must be emphasized that you are not to do anything when you notice any of these four qualities of blocked energy; simply become aware of their existence and take inventory of what and where they are.

Helpful Hints for Awakening Your Chi

Take Your Time

Usually it will take from fifteen minutes to an hour to accomplish what we call awakening the chi. If you feel you have accomplished this in two or three minutes you have definitely not done the exercise correctly.

Internal Scanning Is a Feeling, Not a Visualization Exercise

In doing your internal review, you may not have directly felt your body, but merely visualized or made internal pictures of it, which is an infinitely easier task. You may not like some of the things you *did* feel, but these places will not go away if they are buried or ignored— they must be worked through. You must *allow yourself* to feel the actual state of your insides. You will, over time, gain the power to feel and release your internal blockages.

Let Your Nerves Come Alive

One of the purposes of energy development practice is to promote an entirely new capacity for feeling. The difference in body awareness between a paralyzed person and an average person is as wide as the gap between your present and future state of nerve awareness once your chi practices become established. Do not be frustrated if you cannot feel much at first. Be confident that in time you will be able to feel.

Keep Your Mind Stable

Energy body scanning is not essentially a physical or an intellectual exercise. It is an exercise in specifying, refining and increasing the life-force energies in your body. Small children are known for their short attention spans, but most adults also have what the Chinese call a monkey mind—a mind that cannot be still and jumps from place to place. The mind of those who practice chi develops slowly. Over time, qigong will gradually increase your attention span, concentration and sensitivity to subtle energies.

The Need for Rapid Perfection Slows Progress

It must be understood that this is a process of gradual development. Only the rarest of human beings can do these exercises correctly in the beginning. In the practice of chi development, the more gentle and consistent you are, the faster and steadier your progress will be. Berating yourself will only result in discouragement, even when you are progressing normally. Setting impossible goals and torturing yourself when you do not reach them is a set-up for self-blame and self-sabotage and gets in the way of learning.

Beware of Feelings of Strength

To most people, a sense of strength is a positive and useful thing, something to be valued and sought after. In chi work, however, the feelings of strength are blockages, which prevent the normal, healthy, steady, flow of energy from circulating in a relaxed, powerful fashion.

What Relaxed Chi Feels Like

The ideal is for the energy in any given place in your body to feel relaxed and comfortable, with an easy sense of flow that is full and balanced. You should have a total sense of emptiness connected with your energy. It is only when your energy is blocked that it generates specific feelings.

Lesson 3 The Chi Outer Dissolving Process

Dissolving is the process of fully releasing blocked energy. A classic Taoist metaphor describes the outer dissolving process: ice to water, water to gas. Ice to water more accurately describes the act of sinking your chi; while water to gas is the act of dissolving your chi. Dissolving requires that you work directly with your chi.

Relationship Between Sinking and Dissolving Chi

You can sink your chi without dissolving it. However, you cannot dissolve your chi without also sinking it to some degree. Dissolving is subtler since it works with chi directly; sinking initially works with physical sensations. Each has its strengths, challenges and considerations:

1. Sinking your chi is more accessible and easily learned.

2. Sinking is commonly taught in internal martial arts such as tai chi where acquiring physical power is a main point of competitive success.

3. Sinking builds awareness of the physical sensations in your body that leads to awareness of your chi. Eventually, sinking leads to direct awareness of the chi

that influences your body to become internally wet. This leads to recognizing and directly dissolving blockages in chi during the dissolving process.

4. Learning to sink chi helps to ground you and keep you in the present. It is a safety precaution against disassociating from the emotions that arise when you dissolve and release blocked energy. This is especially important for people who are exceptionally sensitive to chi but rather unconnected to their bodies.

5. Dissolving is more effective and reliable for mitigating and healing disease. Initially, sinking more easily develops chi-generated physical power for martial arts and athletics.

6. At the moment you successfully dissolve your chi, many of the physical sensations that you experienced while sinking your chi will become more pronounced.

7. Eventually, sinking and dissolving will become one seamless process.

8. When either sinking or dissolving you can use your breath to help make you conscious about the subtle layers within a blockage, amplify your awareness or increase your focus. However, do not become too reliant on your breath to accomplish these tasks. You want to be able to sink and dissolve your chi with and without using your breath.

The Etheric Body and Dissolving

There is an energy field that surrounds you called your etheric body or aura. It fluctuates in size based on how strong or weak your chi is from moment to moment, anywhere from six inches to several feet. Dissolving requires you to release energetic blockages within your etheric body to its natural boundary.

All the physical and energetic areas of your physical body are directly connected to corresponding areas within your etheric body. Likewise, blocked areas in your etheric body can directly activate energetic blockages in your physical body and prevent your sinking chi from translating into full resolutions of those blockages.

In dissolving you learn how to release your energy not only downwards but also outwards away from your physical body through your etheric body to its boundary. As you do so, the energy that is released assumes a neutral state and recycles back to you as energy that your physical body can adapt for its ongoing needs.

1. Dissolve Blocked Energy: Ice to Water, Water to Gas

Begin at the crown of your head and notice where you have any feelings of strength, tension, something not being quite right, any general uneasiness or any sense of contraction. These feelings may be physical, energetic, emotional or mental.The blockages that cause these sensations must be dissolved. The dissolving process involves feeling as though these places first change from ice to water and then from water to gas.

2. Dissolve: Shifting from Ice to Water

Once you have identified a place where your energy is blocked or frozen, your awareness should feel the outer contours of this frozen energy. Your awareness will surround and penetrate this solid mass and cause the blockage to soften and allow you to reach its center. This is comparable to what happens when you melt an ice cube: the melting slowly moves from the outside towards the center. You then release the blockage by letting it go *sung*. This is the transformation of ice to water.

3. Dissolve: Transformation of Water to Gas

Once the entire blockage becomes soft and flowing (like an ice cube that has melted and become water), keep your attention on it and have your awareness gently cause the blockage to expand until there is a sense of the trapped energy expanding beyond your body, to where it feels as though it has come to a natural stop or boundary, perhaps as much as a foot or two outside of you. This is the transformation of water to gas.

The dissolving of an energy block moves in stages. At the stage of ice to water, your body will become relaxed, soft and warm as increased chi flow causes your blood circulation to increase. (Remember, your mind moves your chi and your chi moves blood and other fluids.) At the stage of water to gas, pain and the deepest stresses in your body will disappear and, in more advanced qigong, your negative emotions will vanish. You will feel good but the root levels of your energy blockages will not completely disappear.

This dissolving technique must be accomplished by feeling it, not by merely picturing it in your mind's eye. It is a kinesthetic experience.

Relaxation alone may not necessarily result in more energy that can heal your body. You can relax your muscles and still leave emotional blockages untouched. Energetic release affects you on all levels of your being.

At the energetic level although physical relaxation (water) alone makes things temporarily feel better, it alone may only partially release an energy blockage (ice). If because underlying causes of the blockage (ice) have not been dissolved to the boundary of your etheric body, resolved and eliminated (turned to gas), the water can later reconfigure and again return to ice, ultimately resulting in pain or disease.

To get a sense of the dissolving process—ice to water to gas—clench your fist as tight as you can, until your knuckles turn white, which naturally causes your energy to contract. Then put your awareness in your hand and expand your contracted energy until you completely relax your hand (ice to water) without physically opening your fist. Then, continue to focus your awareness on your closed hand until your energy expands out of it into the air and your hand feels that it lacks solidity and is completely amorphous and noncorporeal (water to gas).

4. Standing: Dissolve Downward Through Your Entire Body

A) As you scan inwardly through your body, dissolve an area of blocked energy as completely as possible, until you have an internal sense that it is not possible to dissolve it any further at this time. That is, you reach a point of diminishing returns, where if you were to continue trying to dissolve that point for the next five minutes, five hours, or five years, you would go no further. During the next practice session, you may find that this area feels a little less blocked and is more easily dissolved—whether partially or fully.

B) Next, sink whatever energy remains undissolved down to the second place where energy is bound. Dissolve this combined energy of the first and second places as much as possible. Continuously repeat this procedure as you encounter each new blocked placed further down. You should remember the 70 percent rule. Do not strain by working too hard or dwelling too long on one spot.

C) Sink what remains undissolved down to the third place. Then dissolve the combined energies of the first, second and third places as far as possible. Then continue down in this manner, blockage by blockage, to below your feet.

D) Finally, make a quick pass down your body and release all internal sensations through your feet into the ground, as far down as your awareness continues.

E) Always finish at or below your feet. In order for the energetic clearing you have done during standing to stabilize and not unravel afterwards, you must end each practice at your feet when sinking the chi and below them when scanning and dissolving. If you find that you may run out of time in your pratice before you reach the bottom of your feet, be sure to leave a few minutes at the end to lightly continue down to finish at your feet. This is very important. The longer your practice has been during that session, the more time you should leave at the end to finish well.

The Human Energy Body Expands and Contracts

Your energy body extends below your feet and above your head. Your energy body (etheric body or aura) can grow or shrink many feet, depending upon the vitality or weakness of your internal energy. Some days you may only be able to get your energy an inch into the ground, and other days you may project it many feet. These fluctuations are absolutely normal until your energy body has been developed and stabilized.

Principles Behind the Dissolving Process

The universe is composed of energies that vibrate at different rates. Taoist qigong follows the basic alchemical methodology of raising slow, condensed energetic vibrations, like the physical matter of your body, to more subtle, faster and expansive vibrations, such as emotions and psychic qualities.

The experience of the ancient world, including China, has shown that by focusing concentrated attention, intention and awareness on the energetic aspects of one's being, one is able to raise the potential and actual strength of the body, mind and spirit. This develops physical health, emotional well-being, mental clarity and psychic abilities, ultimately leading to the development of one's spiritual nature and towards becoming one with the nature of the universe: the Tao.

Be Gentle with Yourself

Do not force your chi. Taoism is the path of gentleness, of flowing water. Do not try to push the river. If you have a block you cannot dissolve, go around it and dissolve the rest of your body. Eventually, you will be able to dissolve it—there is absolutely no rush.

Practice Lesson Three for a minimum of two weeks. Then, integrate it into the next level of standing qigong, Opening the Energy Gates of Your Body.

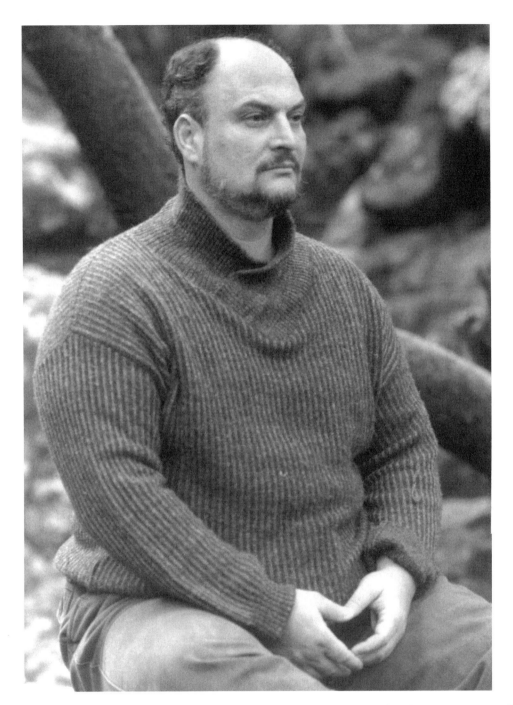

Craig Barnes

Dissolving practices working with the energy gates of the body may be done sitting as well as standing. Beginning practices are generally done with the eyes closed to prevent distraction and keep the student's attention inwards. Once this awareness has stabilized, more advanced practices may be done with the eyes open.

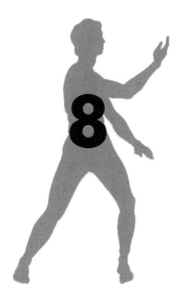

8 Opening the Energy Gates of the Body

What Are the Energy Gates?

The energy gates are major relay stations of the body, where the strength of the life current (chi) moving through the system is regulated. Many gates are located at joints or, more precisely, in the actual space between the bones of a joint. Initially, during your standing and dissolving practice, these are the most important places to clear our blockages.

The concept of "energy gates" is not new; rather, it has been passed down to us from ancient China. Originally worked out by Taoists, it has become common to many traditions. However, to the best of my knowledge, prior to the first publication of this book in 1993, it was never completely described in English.

These gates should not be conceived of as simple anatomical locations. They must be felt with the mind, for they are part of your subtle energy body. From an internal perspective, their locations are approximate and can fluctuate slightly. For acupuncturists, the anatomical location of acupuncture points is valuable, as they utilize these points to put something into the body and use physical markers on the body to get to the approximate location into which a needle is inserted. (The needle indirectly stimulates the body's chi.) Some of the energy gates are the same as the acupuncture points; others are different. The energy gates are like the critical step-up booster stations, each of which controls many smaller power stations.

In qigong the mind is being put directly into the energy gate. You must learn to feel these points in order to channel the flow of your chi to stimulate the subtle body to the greatest extent possible. The object is not merely to visualize the gate (though a knowledge of anatomy can help in locating it), but to feel the gate precisely so you can learn to increase or decrease the amount of power flowing through the gate, using your will or intent with the same amount of ease with which you can now open or shut your eyes, mouth, or hands. Bear in mind that these gates are inside your body and fluctuate minutely in size, depending on the strength of your chi body. Consequently, the exact depth inside the body and the exact location of a gate inside your body at a given point in time is not amenable to visual analysis. The physical and energetic bodies are not identical in form and function, though a good qigong practitioner can feel these energy-gate points in the same manner that other people feel acupuncture needles in their skin. In fact, qigong masters can feel these points in other people as well.

Generally speaking, when we practice "opening" the gates, we will do so in the order given below. Be aware, though, that this order is not written in stone. The most important aspect to remember is that energy and internal sensations always travel *down* the body during the releasing (dissolving) process. The next section explains the locations of the gates to be dissolved.

Important Major and Minor Gates of the Body

When you actually practice the dissolving process, you do not work your way skipping from point to point, energy gate to energy gate, as presented in this book. Rather, you dissolve downwards from the top to the bottom of your body (front, back, and sides simultaneously). The energy gates are points where special attention must be paid as your awareness descends through your body, but anything that is blocked between the energy gates is important and also must be dissolved before moving downward to the next gate. Imagine a great sheet of water descending from the top of your body downwards, dissolving everything in its path. This is how the dissolving process works. This universal energy naturally descends on us every moment, and the important issue is whether or not we can make use of it. This descending "water" is the best defense against burnout from working with the ascending energy or "fire" that emanates from the earth.

Head and Neck

In the beginning, for all the gates of the head, the dissolving process should only reach a depth of half an inch, thereby avoiding the brain. There is a very specific methodology for brain qigong, and it is not a subject for beginners—it should only be studied under the direct supervision of a master.[1] After a month or two of practice it is permissible to dissolve the entire brain at once, but do not dissolve points in the brain separately.

The Crown (Figure 8-1, Gate 1)

The first gate[2] to be dissolved is at the exact center of the crown of the head, which the Chinese call *bai hui*, or the "meeting of a hundred points." At this point, a line drawn over the head from the nose to the cervical spine (neck) would intersect another line drawn from the apex of one ear to the apex of the other.

The Third Eye (Figure 8-1, Gate 2)

Located between the two eyebrows, this point is called the third eye. A person with a history of mental illness should not dissolve this point unless under the supervision of a master. (This gate can open up suppressed areas of a person's psyche, which is best done under the guidance of a qualified master versed in subtleties of the psychic realm.)

The Eyes (Figure 8-1, Gate 3)

This gate is found directly in line with the pupil, just behind the eyeball. This gate is very important for people involved in visually demanding jobs, such as computer operators, as it controls the chi of the visual apparatus and is the interface with the brain. Dissolving this gate can greatly reduce stress that is visually induced.

The Center of the Temples (Figure 8-1, Gate 4)

Usually located on a line from the top of the ear.

The Center of the Ears (Figure 8-1, Gate 5)

The next gate is in the center of the ear, no more than one-quarter of the way into the inner ear. (Except for points along the body's centerline, all gates are found on both sides of the body.)

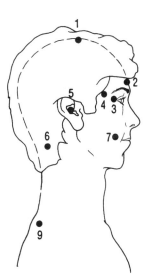

Gates of the Head and Neck
Figure 8-1

---

[1] Specific points in the brain may be felt in qigong practice. Connecting these points energetically in certain configurations can be quite dangerous and can cause serious damage to the brain: other connective configurations can enhance the latent power of the mind. It takes a master with the appropriate knowledge to guide one in this practice.
[2] Remember that the locations of the gates are approximate. The exact locations are to be found by feeling inside your body with your mind.

The Base of the Skull (Figure 8-1, Gate 6)

This point is located at the back of the head, where the spine (atlas vertebra) and skull (occiput) meet. Here, the spinal cord meets the brain stem.

The Roof of the Mouth (Figure 8-1, Gate 7)

This gate is located where the tongue meets the roof of the mouth on the hard palate, where the two main meridians, the governing and conception vessels, join. This gate is where the tongue touches the roof of the mouth.

The Jaw (Figure 8-2, Gate 7a)

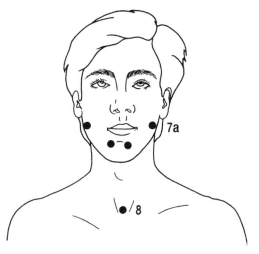

Four Jaw Gates and the Throat Notch
Figure 8-2

There are four minor gates in the jaw that are particularly useful for dealing with TMJ (temporal mandibular joint) problems, jaw tension, and the grinding of teeth. These problems are often results of high-stress conditions. Four points are important for dissolving the jaw: two are at the hinges of the jaw, located at the depression just in front of the lower edge of the ear; the two others are located inside the mouth, on its bottom, behind the front teeth. For the location of these last two gates, imagine lines descending from the inside corner of the eyes down to the bottom to the mouth.

All four of the gates of the jaw should be dissolved simultaneously.

The Throat Notch (Figure 8-2, Gate 8)

The depression just above the breastbone (the sternal notch) is the location of the last major gate of the head and neck.

The Seventh Cervical Vertebra (Figure 8-1, Gate 9)

This gate is found at the big vertebra that usually sticks out at the base of the neck.

Shoulders

The Shoulder Notch (Figure 8-3, Gate 1)

This gate is found at the junction of the acromion and the clavicle, that is, at the end of the collarbone. If the arm is lifted up and to the side, it is where a depression is formed on the top of the shoulder.

The Armpit (Figure 8-3, Gate 2)

This gate is in the center of the armpit, inside the body, about one-third the distance from the skin of the armpit to the shoulder notch. Deeper inside the center of the armpit is another gate connecting all the shoulder gates to the left or right channel.

The Shoulder's Nest (Figure 8-3, Gate 3)

This gate is located in the depression below the outer end of the clavicle (collarbone), lateral to the throat notch. Eventually this area will become soft and pliable, until a depression, or "nest" is formed. Most people are actually very tense and bound up here, so the depression may not be immediately noticeable.

Opening this area dramatically improves flexibility in the arms. This gate is very important for women, because, together with the point in the center of the breast, it

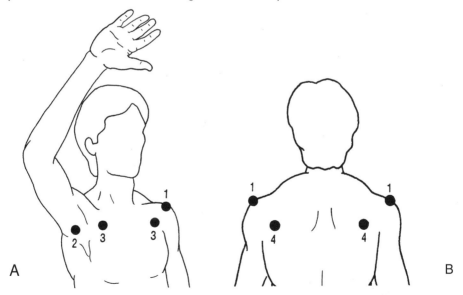

Gates of the Shoulder
A) Anterior gates. B) Posterior gates.
Figure 8-3

regulates the female hormonal system, especially as it affects the breast. In China, these two points are commonly used in qigong treatments for breast problems, including cancer.

The Center of Each Shoulder Blade (Figure 8-3, Gate 4)

This gate is found inside the body in front of the center of the anterior (front) side of each shoulder blade (that is, the side of the shoulder blade that faces the chest).

Arms

Elbow Joint: Back, Inside and Sides—10 Minor Gates; 1 Major Gate (Figure 8-4, Gates 1)

As the elbow, wrist, knee and ankle are the most frequently used joints in the body and must move in many directions, it is important to release the small gates surrounding each of these joints *before* releasing the main gate that is found deep in the center of each of these joints. The gates of the elbow are:

Back: The two indentations just above and the two just below the elbow tip, on either side of the tip (4 minor gates).

Inside: The two indentations just above and the two just below the crease of the elbow, on either side of the tendons (4 minor gates).

Sides: In the center of either side of the elbow (2 minor gates).

Center: Directly in the middle of the elbow joint (1 major gate).

Dissolve each of the back, inside, and side gates of the elbow joint. Then dissolve the center of the joint.

Wrist Joint: Back, Inside and Sides—10 Minor Gates; 1 Major Gate (Figure 8-4, Gates 2)

Back: the two indentations just above and the two just below the back of the

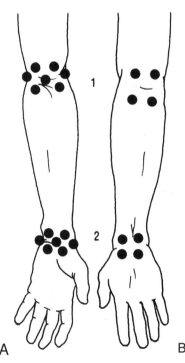

The Elbows and Wrists
(A) Anterior (front) and inside gates.
(B) Posterior (back) gates.
Figure 8-4

wrist joint, on either side of an imaginary line running from the middle finger to the elbow (4 minor gates).

Inside: The two indentations just above and the two just below the crease of the wrist, on either side of the tendons in the center (4 minor gates).

Sides: In the center of either side of the wrist joint (2 minor gates).

Center: In the middle of the wrist joint (1 major gate).

The Carpal and Metacarpal Joints—Illustration Not Shown

Dissolve all the spaces between the small bones in the palm of the hand

The Center of the Palm (Figure 8-5, Gate 4)

The gate in the center of the palm is commonly called the "eye of the hand." Dissolve it. Also dissolve the corresponding gate on the back of the hand. The back-of-the-hand gate is a critical part of the hand for those involved in any form of hands-on energetic healing. Note: It will help to release the center of the palm if you dissolve the space between the palm and the base of the thumb.

The Fingers (Figure 8-5, Gates 5)

In dissolving, pay particular attention to the center of the joints in the fingers.

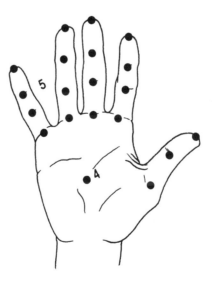

Gates of the Fingers and Palms

Figure 8-5

Complete the dissolving of the fingers by concentrating on the exact center of the fingertips.

Torso

From the Corners of Your Mouth, in a Channel as Wide as Your Mouth, Down the Throat and Sternum to, but Not Including, the Solar Plexus (Figure 8-6)

For the vast majority of the population, the area from where the tongue meets the roof of the mouth, down the throat to just before the solar plexus, is the most difficult for chi to pass through. This region is where the majority of people are blocked up, and it must be completely opened for any chi development practices to progress.[3] Special Note: There are minor energy gates in the joints where the ribs attach to the sternum (breastbone), in the spaces between the ribs around the sides, and in the joints, where ribs attach to the spine *(Figure 8-10)*.

The Center of the Breast (for Women Only) (Figure 8-7, Gate 2)

The breast gates, which have significance only for women, are extremely important for balancing the female hormonal system. These gates, along with those at the shoulder's nest, are commonly used in qigong breast cancer

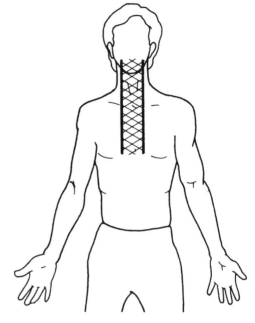

The Channel from the Mouth to the Solar Plexus
Figure 8-6

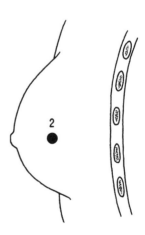

Gate at Center of Breast
Figure 8-7

---

[3] For example, in yoga pranayama, the throat lock is used to open this area.

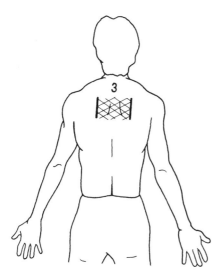

*Many minor energy gates exist in
the area between the shoulder blades.*

Figure 8-8

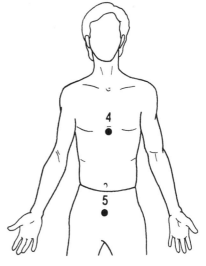

*Gates at Solar Plexus (above)
and Lower Tantien (below).*

Figure 8-9

prevention and treatment in China. These gates are located in the center of each breast, directly behind the nipple in front of the ribs.

Between the Shoulder Blades (Figure 8-8, Gate 3)

Between the shoulder blades and the spine there are a large number of minor energy gates. For athletes, dancers, and martial artists, it is extremely important to open all the gates in this area. The strength of the arms derives in large part from here, while the flexibility of the arms comes mainly from the shoulder's nest.

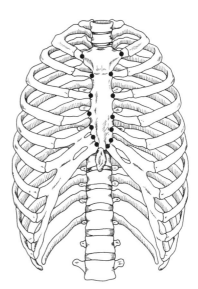

*The Rib Cage. Minor gates at all points
where the ribs attach to the sternum.*

Figure 8-10

Solar Plexus (Figure 8-9, Gate 4)

This gate is located just below the sternum, or breastbone. It is the first soft spot you hit where you tap the middle of the breastbone.

The Lower Tantien and Mingmen (Figure 8-9, Gate 5 and Figure 8-11)

The lower tantien is located in the central core of the body, about two to three inches below the belly button. The mingmen, also known as the "Door of Life," is directly behind the tantien and anterior to (just in front of) the spine.

The tantien is the single most important gate with regard to physical health. Located in approximately the center of the body, all energy lines to physical health and well-being connect here.

The mingmen is an energy point that transfers energy between the spine and the tantien, via a connecting channel inside the abdomen. It is also called the back tantien.

The tantien is the first main focus of all qigong and Taoist alchemical practices. Taoist practices all begin from the premise that physical health is the foundation upon which spiritual development is built, and it is in the lower tantien that all energy affecting the physical body is processed, purified, and generated.

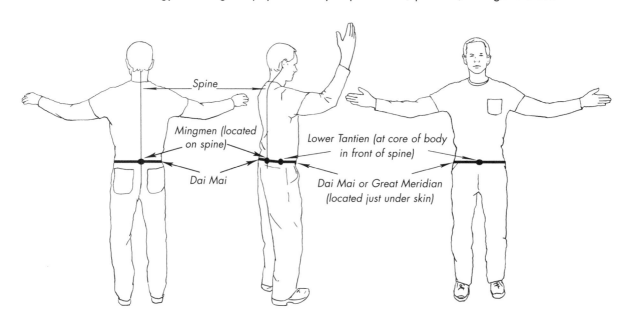

Lower Tantien, Mingmen and Dai Mai
Figure 8-11

This energy can later be connected to the middle and upper tantiens for purposes of emotional and spiritual growth. Martial artists in China who did not have a deep understanding of how to use the lower tantien to purify their grosser emotions merely became very proficient fighting animals.

Eventually, many of the health problems caused by the premature development of the higher psychic centers can be alleviated through practices that involve the lower tantien. For this reason, most of the energy and meditation practices of Japan, China, and Korea, ranging from Zen, to qigong, to the martial arts, pay particular attention to the lower tantien.

Development of the energy in one tantien does not necessarily lead to development of the others. We have all met people who are physically healthy and emotional, psychic or spiritual wrecks. It is also common for people who are advanced on the emotional, psychic or spiritual planes to have incredible health problems. This is often because the energy of the higher centers is creating more energetic pressure than the body can handle.

Many people in the Zen community, for instance, develop bad health problems from meditation. Even the enlightened Japanese Zen master Hakuin had to go to a Taoist to repair the damage he had done to his body by prolonged sitting.

Chan Buddhism, the precursor to Zen, had a very strong qigong component to its practices, which was lost when Chan techniques were introduced from China to Japan. In Tibetan Buddhism, the initial 100,000 prostrations *(nundro)* have the function of developing the body before a practitioner gets into the more psychic aspects of the teachings. Yogis in India, Tibet, and China usually do some sort of physical and energetic practices to maintain the health of their bodies during their multiyear retreats, or else risk health problems.

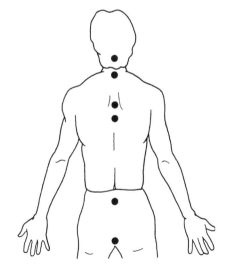

Major Gates of the Spine
Figure 8-12

Back Muscles—Illustration Not Shown

Dissolve all the energy in the back muscles, especially the energy around the kidneys. Begin from the neck and shoulder area and work slowly downwards to the top of the buttocks.

Spine (Figure 8-12)

Beginning at the base of the skull, dissolve the entire spine, especially between the vertebrae. Pay special attention to the following locations: the place where the spine enters the skull; the big vertebra at the base of the neck; the vertebra between the shoulder blades; the vertebra just below the shoulder blades; the vertebra level with mingmen; and the tailbone.

Pelvis

The Pelvic Girdle (Figure 8-13)

Dissolve the bones that make up the pelvic girdle; that is, the ilium, ischium, sacrum, and coccyx (tailbone), especially the places where they join.

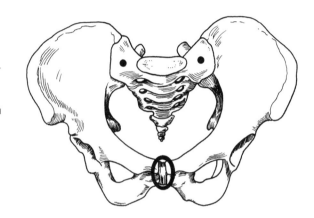

Gates of the Pelvis
Figure 8-13

The Hip Socket, or Acetabulum (between the Head of the Thigh Bone and the Hip Socket)—Illustration Not Shown.

The Area Inside the Pelvis, Starting from the Crest of the Hip Bones All the Way Through to the Inguinal Crease (Kwa)—Illustration Not Shown

The Genitals—Illustration Not Shown

Women should dissolve the whole vaginal canal up to the cervix, but not the cervix itself. There is an energetic wall at the cervix that separates the womb from the vagina, and this should not be dissolved.[4] Men should practice the dissolving

---

[4]Dissolving the cervix area excessively can disrupt a women's reproductive energy and may subsequently lead to menstrual problems, PMS, vaginal infections, and the inability to conceive. This natural energetic seal should be broken only at childbirth. It is also possible to dissolve the womb, but excessive practice can make a woman more fertile—an important issue in this era of birth control.

procedure from the prostrate and down the shaft of the penis, as well as from the prostrate to the testicles.

The Anus and Rectum—Ilustration Not Shown

Dissolve from as far up the anus as any blockage is felt, but generally no more than an inch or two. This is an extremely important gate, and is definitely helpful in relieving constipation, hemorrhoids, and preventing colon cancer.

The Perineum—Illustration Not Shown

Located between the genitals and the anus, the perineum is the point where energy from the legs and the body joins.

Legs

The legs and buttocks support the spine, both physically and energetically

Knee Joint: Front, Back and Sides—10 Minor Gates; 1 Major Gate (Figure 8-14 and Figure 8-15)

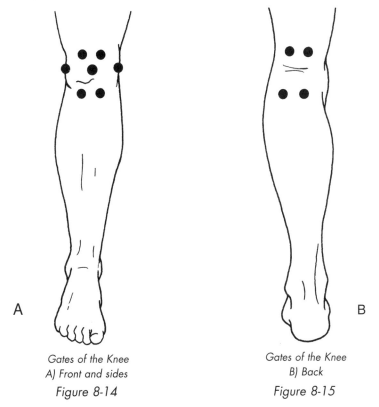

A

Gates of the Knee
A) Front and sides
Figure 8-14

B

Gates of the Knee
B) Back
Figure 8-15

Front: The eyes of the knee; that is, the two indentations just above and below the middle of the kneecap, on either side of its centerline (4 minor gates).

Back: Beneath the tendons on either side of the back of the knee, above and below the crease (4 minor gates).

Sides: In the center of either side of the knee (2 minor gates).

Center: Directly in the middle of the knee joint (1 minor gate).

Ankle Joint: Front, Back, and Sides—8 Minor Gates; 1 Major Gate (Figure 8-16, Gates 2 and Figure 8-17, Gates 2)

Front: Just above and below the crease formed by pulling the foot up, on either side of the centerline of the shin bone (4 minor gates).

Back: Just above the point of insertion of the Achilles tendon into the heel bone, on either side (2 minor gates).

Sides: In the center of the ankle bone on either side (2 minor gates).

Center: Directly in the middle of the ankle joint (1 major gate).

The Tarsals and Metatarsals—Illustration Not Shown

Dissolve all the spaces between the small bones of the foot.

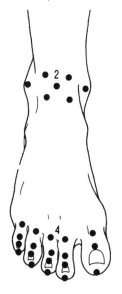

Gates of the Ankles and Toes

Figure 8-16

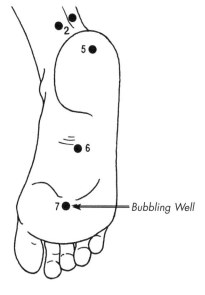

Major Gates of the Bottom of the Foot and the Back of the Ankle

Figure 8-17

The Toes (Figure 8-16, Gates 4)

Dissolve all the toe joints, up to and especially including the tips of the toes.

The Heel (Figure 8-17, Gate 5)

About one inch from the very back of the foot, on the centerline of the foot.

The Arch (Figure 8-17, Gate 6)

In the center of the arch, on the midline of the foot (inside the foot).

The Bubbling Well (Figure 8-17, Gate 7)

About one quarter of the distance from the base of the toes to the heel, on the bottom of the foot. This gate is in the center of the depression formed in the ball of the foot when you point your toes.

Below the Feet and Above the Head

Your energetic body extends below your feet and above your head. The size of your energetic body, unlike your physical body, grows and shrinks with time. It is in constant flux. Over time, and with practice, your energy body will grow in size and strength, but it will still fluctuate.

Feel below your body until you cannot feel anymore and you find where your energy body has reached its natural end. Dissolve the energy from the bottom of your feet downward until the energy ends. No matter in what environment you find yourself, always dissolve to the ends of your energy body.

Your energy body also ends above your head. (Some of the Yoga traditions refer to the eighth and ninth chakras, located above your head.)

Feel above your head until the sense of energy ends (see p. 124 and p. 238). This is where you will now begin all dissolving practices. One complete standing exercise will constitute dissolving the energy from above the head, through the body, and culminate with all the energy dissolving into the energy point below your feet, that is, your root. After standing, open your eyes slowly, making sure that you do not jar the comfortable relaxed feeling you had when your eyes were closed.

Opening the Gates: A Lesson Plan

Each lesson should be practiced for at least three days, or as long as you need to stabilize the gate or gates referred to in the lesson. Moving too fast creates strain and scatters energy, resulting in little benefit.

First, lightly dissolve all energy gates you have previously opened, and then spend the remaining 80 percent of your practice time on opening the next set of gates below. It is important to dissolve all the blocked energy above these new gates; this includes not just the energy that is blocked at the major gates, but energy blocked anywhere else as well. For example, when moving from the crown to the third eye, be sure to dissolve the forehead, and when moving from the hips to the knees be sure to dissolve the thighs.

If you feel that too much material is contained in one lesson, just divide it up. Go at your own pace—there is no pressure to complete this process in any specific amount of time. Generally speaking, allow at least one to three months to work your way down through all the gates to your feet.

At the end of any practice session, gently dissolve through the rest of the body to the floor. Suggested lessons for dissolving (each number consists of one lesson) are below.

1. Bai hui, or the crown of the head.
2. The third eye, the eyes, the center of the ears, and the temple. Also, the four jaw points.
3. Where the tongue touches the roof of the mouth and the throat notch.
4. The base of the skull and in between each of the cervical (neck) vertebrae down to the seventh cervical vertebra at the base of the   neck.
5. From where the tongue touches the roof of your mouth to the end of the breastbone, on a line about the width of your mouth.
6. The four points of the shoulder.
7. The elbows.
8. The wrists.
9. The hands (all the points).
10. The joints where the ribs connect to the sternum, the spaces between the ribs, the joints where the ribs connect to the spine, the area between the shoulder blades and the spine. For women only: the gates of the breasts (directly behind the nipples).

11. The solar plexus.
12. The whole of the belly, starting from the front and dissolving through the internal organs back to the spine.
13. The tantien and the mingmen.
14. All the points along the spine, from the occiput to the tailbone, paying special attention to the occiput, the seventh cervical vertebra, the vertebra in the center of the shoulder blades, the one at the base of the shoulder blades, mingmen and the tailbone.
15. The hip sockets, the pelvic bones, and the kwa (that is, the area inside the front crest of the hip bones).
16. The anus.
17. The genitals.
18. The perineum.
19. The knees.
20. The ankles.
21. The feet.
22. Below the floor.
23. Above the head.

After completing this sequence, begin all further standing qigong from above the head, and dissolve down the body one level at a time. Imagine the body to be full of water, with the water being slowly let out from the bottom of your feet. As the water level drops, dissolve everything at the new level—front, back, and sides.

When dissolving the crown of the head, you want to dissolve everything else at the same level; that is, the entire tip of your head. As you work towards the next gate, the third eye, dissolve down the head so that all sides of the head at the same level are dissolved simultaneously. At the solar plexus, then, you would also be working on all the body parts that are located approximately at the same level, i.e., the lower ribs, those vertebrae at the level of the lower ribs, and the elbows.

Guidelines for Practicing Standing Qigong

1. Don't Overstrain Your Energy System

Release as much as possible of the blocked (stuck) energy above the gate you are working on and drop what remains into the next lower gate. Continue on down through successive lower gates to below the floor. Spend three or four days until the mind has become reasonably stable there. Work slowly on each gate (or series of gates), releasing enough energy above each new gate so that energy can be released from the gate itself without overstraining the system. If you go too fast, it creates strain, energy is scattered and little progress is made.

2. Dissolve from the Skin Inward

In general, begin on the outer surface of the body, and over the next months begin to go deeper and deeper, until eventually you gain a direct experience of the bones. Also, remember that during the first month or two, you should not go more than one-half inch into the brain, though later it is permissible to extend the dissolving process through the entire brain. Just be sure not to do anything specific with the chi of gates you encounter inside the brain, such as making connections or geometric patterns.

3. Allow Six Months to Stabilize the Tantien and Mingmen

Moving down through the gates of the body to the tantien will usually take at least a month, it will probably be another month before the tantien stabilizes (fixes in location), and it will take anywhere from three to six months before you will be able to extend your mind from the tantien (in the center) to the mingmen (on the spine). It will also take three to six months to begin to store energy in the tantien. This process can be accelerated when studying with a master, and may take longer on your own.

4. The Legs Are More Difficult than the Arms

In general, especially for Westerners, the legs will be more difficult to open than the arms, as in the West we tend to focus on our heads and upper bodies. Also, we do not tend to sit or squat on the floor. Because Westerners do not tend to direct chi into their legs, the legs become insensitive to energy.

5. Stand for a Minimum of Five Minutes to Get Benefits

As a general rule, a minimum of five minutes of standing is necessary for any noticeable results. This presupposes that a person is able to drop into a state of complete relaxation in thirty or forty seconds, and after a few months of practice this is a highly realistic goal. In the beginning, however, it may take five minutes to attain a reasonable state of relaxation. If this is so, those five minutes must be added to the practice time; in other words, ten minutes would be necessary for any benefit to accrue. On a super-stressed day, you might require fifteen minutes just to relax enough to begin the standing practice.

The longest I have seen people do standing and still gain benefit from it is about six hours at a time. Usually they are still in their teens or their twenties and have little stress or work pressures. For the average person, standing beyond one hour at a time usually is impractical, and therefore one hour can be considered a maximum practice time. To reach this amount, gradually increase the length of practice by two or three minutes every day, or even every week or month.

If you can only practice five, ten or fifteen minutes a day during the week and then do an hour or two on the weekend, your muscles may become sore. A half an hour might be called for, but not much more until you have built up to it. Never strain yourself internally. Slow, steady, even, and with moderation should be the key guidelines for the average person who wants to maintain or improve health, flexibility, and well-being. Of course, these principles also apply to martial artists and athletes, but what is moderate for them, the average person would no doubt find somewhat excessive.

6. Standing for People Involved in Movement Arts

Since the movement arts require superior flexibility and body control, people involved in these arts should do a minimum of twenty minutes standing at a time, up to a maximum of two hours or more, depending upon how strong they want their energy to be and how deeply they desire mastery and knowledge of their physical being. Practicing in this range will take one beyond mere physical maintenance to a level of superior physical ability. For those under 25, the amount of practice time could quite possibly be increased, whereas those over 50 might want to start with a little less.

Always bear in mind never to overstrain, as this can create an internal resistance to practicing. If the body or mind is pushed too far in one direction it will naturally snap back in the other direction. Consistent practice will get you much further than periodic blasts, which often cause your practice time afterwards to dramatically diminish. A two-and-a-half hour marathon could be so internally exhausting that the internal resistance to further exhaustion would prevent practice for the next week or so.

7. Standing for Martial Artists and Healers

Martial artists should be aware that the standing posture has been used in China for thousands of years to develop internal power. At more advanced stages, there are many hand postures that open up every energy line in the body and allow the manifestation of internal power from any part of the body at will. As part of both internal martial arts and traditional Chinese healing and bodywork (qigong tui na), there are approximately 200 different hand postures (see Chapter 15), each with different mind components, which are capable of developing internal power and healing the damage caused by illness and injury. Each of these postures deals with a specific way in which energy is not moving through the system. With practice, it is possible to make energy move through any blockage in the system, whether in internal organs, nerve tissue, soft tissue, or the spine.

When I was younger I practiced six hours at a stretch in order to increase my internal power. At that time I was actively involved in fighting competitions where it was easy to get severely hurt, and this significantly increased my motivation to learn. If I did not practice hard enough, I was realistically looking at an opponent putting me in the hospital. Most people do not have this strong motivation, and the majority of people practicing the internal martial arts are not in their late teens and early twenties. Therefore, I would say that between one and three hours a day is the maximum that the average dedicated martial artist or healer should be practicing.

8. Do Not Stand Too Long

It is important to realize that there is a point of diminishing returns, beyond which the extra practice doesn't really result in enough benefit to be worth it. Again, beware of the internal exhaustion factor: If you get too internally exhausted, you will not be able to practice for days. So find where this maximum benefit point is for you and, keeping in mind the 70 percent rule, don't go beyond it. It is normal to learn through the school of hard knocks where your limits are. Internal exhaustion is infinitely more tiring than exhaustion attained through external exercise, including marathon running—it is like nervous exhaustion combined with physical exhaustion.

9. Dissolve Your Energy Blocks at Progressively Deeper Levels

The average practice period consists of a period of settling in, followed by a period where everything feels wrong and you begin concentrating on the weakest (most obviously bound-up) link in your chain. Then, after feeling like you've unknotted that block, a tremendous sense of liberated energy is felt moving within. The point at which this liberated energy begins to weaken is when most people call it a day.

However, after much practice (months to years), it is possible to find a second weak link, dissolve it, and get a new burst of energy. Only the most experienced practitioners can go through this cycle three or four times, and these people are rare.

Again, the keys to success are consistency and not overdoing it. If these are adhered to, standing can give a martial artist or athlete an easy, relaxed, and effortless power that cannot be gained through any amount of physical training or weightlifting.

10. Always Finish At the Bottom of Your Feet or Energy Body

Coordinating Your Breath with Qigong Movements

The chapters you have read so far have covered standing practices in detail and have described the basics of Longevity Breathing. Chapters 9-14 teach the movements of Opening the Energy Gates Qigong.

When physical movements of qigong are coordinated with breathing, it increases your chi. This practice can be either good or bad, and while some qigong and tai chi schools advocate it, some do not.

The classical Taoist position is that it is good to strengthen the breath under all conditions but not to coordinate inhales and exhales with physical movements in the beginning stages of qigong practice.

The chi that energizes your body and energy channels can simultaneously charge up your emotions. If your basic emotional predisposition is to be positive, happy or calm, more chi will provide you the energy to be happier, calmer and more positive. If the opposite is true more chi can turn you more negative and release your inner demons. Thus, there is the possibility that the stronger one becomes physically, the more likely that one may develop into an emotional wreck. Many people in the sports and martial arts community have suffered on this account: they becomes aware of the physical, but not the emotional (or psychic) level of chi.

Breath and Emotions

Thoughts and emotions create "waves" in the mind. The way one breathes can create these waves and cause the mind to take on the thought wave pattern of specific emotions. For example, when you get angry, your breath rises to your chest, and then to your head with short, powerful bursts. Conversely, if you start breathing from the chest and head intentionally with short, powerful bursts, you will start feeling angry. On the other hand, if you are feeling depressed, which usually results in very shallow breathing, and you consciously start deep, regular breathing, you will feel less depressed. You can change or at least mask your true feelings with your breath.

Usually when the breath and the mind are coordinated, one simply experiences the emotion. However, if you practice the qigong method of coordinating the physical breath with specific body movements, you may cause emotional suppression to occur. You may only become more aware of your breath and movement and not your emotions. The artificial breathing pattern masks awareness of your actual emotions, and at the same time, you strengthen these invisible emotions by your practice. Coordinating breath with movement will increase your physical capacities and charge up your physical chi, but it may also charge up the deeper layers of your being, the emotional and psychic basement where the emotions reside that have been repressed over a lifetime.

There is also the possibility that emotional energy may be increased when you coordinate your breath with movements. If, for example, you are already angry or depressed and aren't even aware that you are, you could find yourself becoming extremely explosive or even more overtly depressed without knowing why.

Dealing with Negative Emotions

The goal of many Taoist energy exercises is to make you aware of negative emotions and give you the tools to dissipate them. However, by coordinating your breathing with your movements in the initial learning stages, you may actually strengthen them and lock them in more strongly.

The better way to deal with negative emotion is as follows: As you stand, become aware of your negative emotions and notice what they feel like. Recognize how they create physical tension in your body and changes in your mood. Then relax and release the tension by using the dissolving methods explained in Chapter 7 to whatever extent is possible. Do not suppress the feelings that arise.

Repeat the same process while moving. Initially, do not consciously coordinate the extensions and retractions of your arms and legs with inhaling and exhaling. After you have the experience to recognize how and if emotions are being activated, and you can relax, dissolve and let go of them, you can then breathe in coordination with your movements and simultaneously release your emotions.

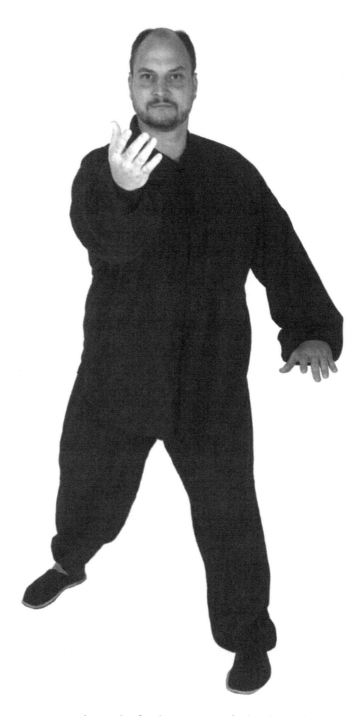

Anthony Ortega

Bruce Frantzis shows the final extension of Cloud Hands.

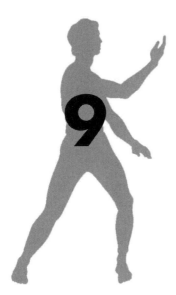

9 Cloud Hands: Rooting the Lower Body

Cloud Hands Is the Most Complete Qigong Movement

Cloud Hands contains all the same essential energy elements that make tai chi chuan the highly effective system of healing that it is. If you could only practice one single move for health, Cloud Hands would be it. It involves both the arms and the legs in forward, backward, upward and downward movements. Cloud Hands includes all tai chi's basic twisting, turning, bending, and stretching motions, and begins the process of lengthening the tissues of the body. Although there is no shifting of the weight forward and back, the weight does shift completely from one side to the other, and thus Cloud Hands contains the basic process of moving from empty to full, that is, one leg becomes empty (of weight) as the other becomes full. The principles learned in Cloud Hands also apply to hsing-i, bagua and the vast majority of qigong and neigong exercises.

In the different styles of tai chi chuan, Cloud Hands is performed in many different ways. The Cloud Hands described here is fairly simple, and derives from an original Taoist practice that contains all the internal principles (without necessarily the specific form) of the Yang, Wu, Chen, and combination tai chi/hsing-i/bagua styles.

Beginning with the feet and working up to the hands, this exercise will be taught in a number of stages, each of which incorporates essential internal principles.

Transition from Standing and Dissolving to Cloud Hands

Gently Open Your Eyes

When you are standing with your eyes closed and dissolving internal blockages, it is quite natural to go into a light trance. In time, this light trance state will pass, as internal clarity becomes stronger. In the beginning, however, it is normal to slow down and become extremely relaxed.

Cloud Hands is done with the eyes open. After standing, slowly open your eyes, making sure that your entrance into the world of sight is a gradual and comfortable one. In order to do this, open your eyes at the same internal speed that you have previously been experiencing your insides with eyes closed. The object is to have a smooth transition from internal awareness to external awareness, avoiding a shock similar to that which individuals would experience if they were to come from a dark cave and suddenly open their eyes to bright sunlight, or cold water were thrown on them while in a deep sleep. Maintaining the relaxation and internal sense of openness experienced in standing as you transit into moving allows you to carry over this relaxation into movement. Thus the movement can increase relaxation and develop even more energy.

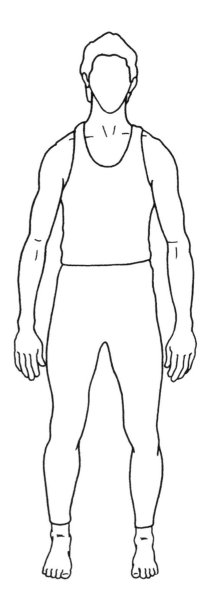

Standing Posture. Feet are parallel, shoulder-width apart.

Figure 9-1

Lesson 1 Root the Lower Body

1. Place your feet parallel to each other, shoulder-width apart *(Figure 9-1)*.

2. With your eyes open and your feet parallel, shift all your weight (100 percent) to your weaker leg, let's say the left. Keeping the weight there, extend your right leg to the side a few inches, maintaining both feet parallel *(Figure. 9-2A)*. Keep the weight of the weighted foot (in this case, the left) evenly distributed, so that no one part of the foot has any more or less weight than any other.

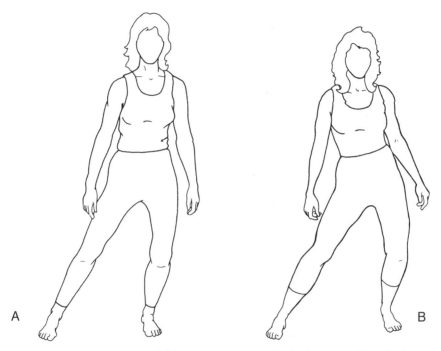

Weight 100 percent on left leg. A) Correct: Hips level. B) Incorrect: Hips tilted.
Figure 9-2

3. Then extend your energy and your weight through your feet to the point below the floor where your energy body ends; this is your root. If you are able to extend your energy below the floor, the energy of the earth will naturally connect with your body's energy. You will then be able to draw energy into your body from the earth just as a tree does, as well as circulate chi from the right to the left side of your body and from left to right when you shift weight to the opposite foot.

Lesson 2 Point Your Tailbone Down and Slowly Shift Weight

Check that your tailbone is pointed to the ground and your spine is straight.

1. Shift Weight

Shift your weight 100 percent from left leg to right leg, and right leg to left leg, back and forth, a number of times. (Most people will find that their leg muscles will ache after a while; this is only natural.) The shifting must be slow and steady, and as far as possible free of any jerks or spasms, and speed should remain constant throughout the shift. Check that your hips remain even, parallel to the floor, and are not shifting up or down with the movement *(Figure 9-3A)*.

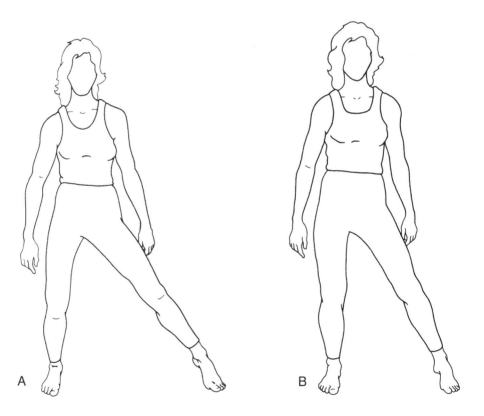

The 70 percent rule. A) Leg width is at 100 percent of capacity. B) Leg width brought back to 70 percent of capacity.

Figure 9-3

2. The 70 Percent Rule (as Applied to Leg Width)

The first question that often comes to mind has to do with how far apart to put the legs. Again we come to a fundamental principle concerning how these, and all Taoist exercises, are done: the 70 percent rule. In any tai chi or qigong exercise, first estimate what 100 percent of your physical capacity is in terms of range of movement or time of practice; in this case, how far your legs can comfortably widen. Once you determine this, you then only move or practice to approximately 70 percent of your capacity *(Figure 9-3B)*. This percentage is not rigid, and the appropriate amount could be anywhere from 60 percent to 80 percent, depending on your condition.

If people were totally sensitive and aware of all their internal limitations, there probably would not be much need to mention this rule. The principle upon which the 70 percent rule is based is that development must begin by considering your weakest link. Do not seek maximum performance, as that quest may both damage the weak link and cause the whole system to contract and tense up.

3. Use A Partner to Practice With

You will find it very helpful to practice the weight-shifting motion with one or two other people. In this particular exercise, have one person check that your lower back is straight, and the other person watch that your hips move from side to side without going up and down. Also, have your partner make sure that your body does not rise and fall as you shift your weight from side to side. Make sure that both feet are completely flat on the floor (except the arch, of course), and that all parts of the sole of the foot touch the floor equally. The weight should not ride on the inner or outer edge of the foot, forward on the ball of the foot, or backward on the heel.

Important Points to Remember

1. The "Give 100 Percent" Attitude Can Be Dangerous

Stay within your approximately 70 percent capacity. Commonly, when people try to give 100 percent, they inadvertently go to 110 or 120 percent of their body's maximum capacity, which results in injury, sometimes slight and sometimes severe. We've all heard of the beginning runner who goes out on his first day knowing he needs to warm up. He stretches his legs, starts running, reaches 100 percent of his capacity without knowing it, and when he decides to go a little further ("more is better") he pulls his

hamstring. Three weeks later he tries again, maybe a little wiser, but most likely not.

Another factor is at work here. At 70 percent of your perceived performance level, you can throw 100 percent of your energy and effort into developing what you are practicing. Yet as you approach 100 percent of capacity, the body will subconsciously react with fear to potential damage. This fear is a necessary and natural survival mechanism, and even without your awareness, your body and mind will tense up in response to it. Since two of the fundamental purposes of the core exercises are to develop deep relaxation and reduce stress in the body, this 100 percent attitude is counterproductive.

Many athletes will overtrain to win, resulting in permanent damage to their bodies. This is opposite to the principles of the Opening the Energy Gates exercises, which aim to make your body and mind work in a more relaxed, efficient and healthy manner for the rest of your life. The more you practice them, the more energy you have—so long as you keep within the 70 percent rule. The 70 percent rule prevents people from becoming heroes at the expense of their bodies.

2. Moderation Protects Old Injuries

Many people with weak knees, bad ankles, back problems or old injuries (which they may even be unaware of), will find that keeping to this principle of moderation will save a lot of physical pain and bodily damage, whether doing qigong or any other type of exercise. The majority of Westerners do not have a regular exercise regimen, and therefore try to do everything in the first week, or even the first day. The one thing all athletes understand is that you often do not know what injuries have occurred until the next day. The purpose of the 70 percent rule is to prevent injuries before they occur.

It has been my experience, having taught thousands of people, that many people ignore these safety warnings even after several injuries! It is my hope that you will re-read the 70 percent rule at least three or four times, and take note of when your body speaks to you (see p. 28). It would prefer that you did not damage it.

Mechanics of the Joints

The fundamental structure of a human joint is a ball and socket. A ball and socket is like a mortar and pestle, and, as with a mortar and pestle, the object is to squeeze or grind up the contents contained and not the container.

Human joints, likewise, are not designed to have the ball grind on the socket. In the joints, there is a substance called synovial fluid, which is capable of tremendous compression. This fluid acts as a buffer between the ball and the socket, and compresses and expands in proportion to the amount of pressure put on it.

One basic function of muscles is to keep the alignment of the bones in a joint stable, so that the joint's natural hydraulic abilities can manifest. If the ball and the socket fit evenly into each other, the joint will receive a bare minimum of shock no matter what action is performed.

Human beings were meant to be able to walk on their legs for 70 to 80 years. They were meant to be able to move things with their arms millions of times in a lifetime. Your joints will not wear out if the internal pressure of the synovial fluid is kept constant and if the ball and socket joints remain aligned. However, if the proper alignment is lost, the ball can slowly damage the socket, or vice versa. The supporting ligaments, muscles, and tendons can become overstretched or damaged, resulting in further misalignment. This vicious cycle causes the joints to weaken and lose their natural capacity to function. Thus, a person can eventually become arthritic or too weak to do even the simplest tasks.

Negative Effects of Joint Problems on the Whole Body

According to Chinese medical thinking and the science of chi development, when problems begin in a joint, energy begins to stagnate there, so that it cannot circulate to the rest of the system. This situation causes a number of extremely negative effects. First of all, local blood circulation is decreased, which then decreases the circulation throughout the body. Secondly, as the chi or energy of the body stagnates in the joint, the internal organs do not receive as much energy as they need. Thirdly, though the joint has plenty of coagulated energy, it is still starved of good energy, and it thus begins to pull energy from healthy tissues of the body, thereby weakening those tissues.

The sequence of the weakening of the tissues is: The stagnated joints pull energy from other joints, then from the organs, then from the spine, and then from the brain. So one of the first goals of qigong is to release bound-up joints; then energy can flow smoothly through the system.

Proper Alignment of the Knee Joint

Both in standing and in the initial movement from side to side, make sure that all parts of your foot (aside from the arch) are touching the floor equally. When one part of your foot rises or collapses, this is a clear sign that the ankle joint is not aligned. Also check to make sure that your knee joint is aligned with your ankle *(Figures 9-4A and B)*. It is the shin that connects your knee to your ankle. In order for this connection to be solid, with the legs slightly bent, the internal line from the center of the knee to the center of the ankle in the weight-bearing leg must be stable and directly connected, at a 90° angle to the floor. When viewed from the front, a vertical line dropped from the center of your patella (kneecap) directly downwards should go through the center of your foot. Under no circumstances should a beginner have the front of the knee extend beyond the tips of the toes.

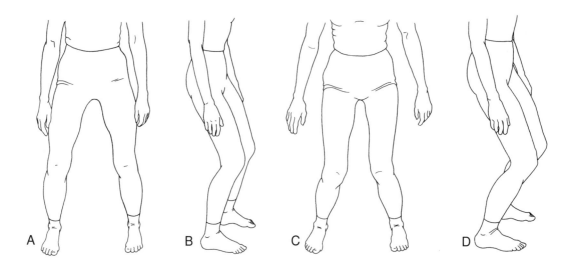

Knee Alignment. A) and B) Correct: Center of knee above center of foot.
C) Incorrect: Knees collapsed inward. D) Incorrect: Knees collapsed forward.

Figure 9-4

The Knee Is a Weight-Transference Joint, Not a Weight-Bearing Joint

An extension of the above consideration is that if someone were to push downwards on the crest of the hip from the side of your body, the alignment of the body should be such that the pressure goes directly into the center of the arch of the foot. No pressure should be felt in the knee joints—the knee should be a weight-transference joint, not a weight-bearing joint.

When the knee joint is properly aligned, there is a feeling of tremendous springiness, not unlike that felt when using a bicycle pump or pushing on the brakes of a car. This springiness does not require any physical exertion, as the alignment itself will create the springiness.

Two-Person Exercise to Test the Alignment of the Knee Joint

Here is a simple exercise to help you acquire the sensation of a properly aligned knee joint. Have a partner gently push down on your thigh and into your knee as you shift from side to side. This will lead to the discovery that only one or two of the many possible positions of your knee and ankle will be comfortable and stable. Don't push with so great a force as to risk injury; the object is purely to find where the knee and ankle alignment is stable and springy.

Practice going from side to side with a partner until both of you are able to recognize the proper joint alignment. Remember to find this alignment whenever you practice internal energy exercises of any nature, or, for that matter, any normal athletic activities. This particular technique generally makes a huge difference to golfers, weightlifters, skiers and participants in other sports where tremendous pressure is exerted on the knees and ankles.

Importance of Opening the Back of the Knee Joint

Other knee problems suffered by all sorts of athletes, as well as qigong and tai chi practitioners, are caused by not properly opening up the back of the knee. Most people bend their knees in such a way as to put all the stress into the front of the knee, which structurally is very weak. The back of the knee closes while the front of the knee opens, creating a very small "V" shape. The pressure on the front of the knee slowly pulls out some of the soft tissue (ligaments, muscles, tendons) and creates knee problems. This can be thought of as a self-inflicted knee lock, functioning just like a martial arts wrist lock or elbow twist.

Two-Person Exercise to Align the Knee and Ankle Joints

Here is another helpful exercise to align the joints of the knees and ankles. Working with a partner, lie on the floor and lift one leg up to chest height. Your partner grabs the heel and ball of your foot and pushes forward (not hard). You must discover the alignment of the

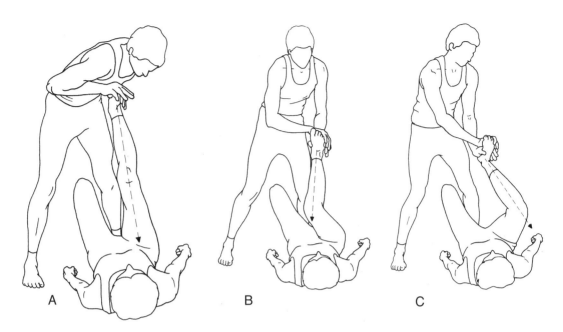

Aligning the Knee and Ankle Joints. A) Correct: Hip, knee, and ankle joints in a line.
B) Incorrect: Knee collapsed inward. C) Incorrect: Knee turned outward.

Figure 9-5

knee, ankle, and kwa, which uses the natural pressure of the synovial fluid, to push back with the bare minimum of effort *(Figure 9-5A)*. Rely on the springiness of the joint, rather than the muscles. If the joint is not aligned properly, the experience will be one of muscle strain and discomfort, and if the joint is really out of line, there will also be pain. If, however, the foot, ankle, knee, and kwa are properly aligned, you will be able effortlessly to push several people away from you with your leg.

If you have had any back, knee, or ankle injuries, be very gentle throughout these exercises, as you are only trying to find the difference between the ease and comfort of a properly aligned joint, and the strain and discomfort of an improperly aligned one. Human beings, barring accidents or genetic problems, were designed to be able to walk for many miles without great effort. With these exercises, you are simply becoming conscious of the natural mechanisms that allow the body to function optimally.

Lesson 3 Opening and Closing the Kwa

What Is the Kwa?

Included within the kwa area are: 1) the left and right channels of the energy; 2) the pelvis, including the hip joint: 3) the sacrum and first few lumbar vertebrae; 4) the iliopsoas muscle group; 5) the adductor muscles; 6) the pelvic diaphragms (the health of which is essential to sexual vitality); 7) the lower intestine; and 8) the rectum.

The muscles of the kwa *(Figure 9-6)* connect the legs to the spine: the iliopsoas connects the lumbar vertebrae to the pelvis and femur (thigh bone), and the adductors connect the pelvis to the femur. The springiness of the spine and legs is partially determined by the elasticity of the iliopsoas muscles. Many lower back problems are caused by stiffness, spasm, or trauma in the iliopsoas muscles.

At the inguinal groove, the largest collection of lymph nodes in the body can be found. Lymph is a critical component of the body's immune response system. Unlike blood, which is moved by the heart and vascular system, lymph is basically moved by muscular contractions. Nature is very wise—every time we walk or move our legs and arms, large lymph collectors (at the inguinal groove, or the armpits, for example) are activated, thus moving our lymph. Chinese neigong exercises simply increase this natural phenomenon, thereby strengthening a very important component of the immune system. Increasing the movement of the internal elements of the kwa is one of the most significant and unique contributions to the health effects of all chi-enhancing body practices.

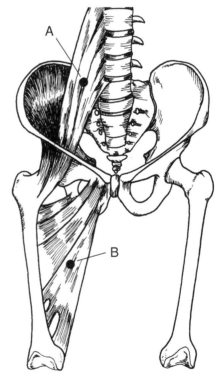

Deep Muscles of the Kwa.
A) Iliopsoas group. B) Adductor group.
Figure 9-6

1. Assume the Basic Standing Posture

Make sure you maintain all the proper structural alignments. Be especially careful to align the knees and ankle, with all points of your foot touching the floor evenly. Check the alignment by sinking your hips to see if you can feel your hips directly pressing on the arch of your foot. All weight and pressure should transfer through your knee and ankle joints to the foot. Bounce lightly, using your hips so that you can feel the spring in your legs.

For this lesson, the knees must remain fixed in space, moving neither forward nor backward, whether going up or down. This can be checked in several ways: have a partner position his or her arm in front of your kneecaps, or use a chair or piece of string. It is important that, whatever feedback method you choose, you do not use a rigid or immovable object like a wall or a heavy piece of furniture. You want to find out if your kneecaps are moving in space, but you don't want to put pressure on them.

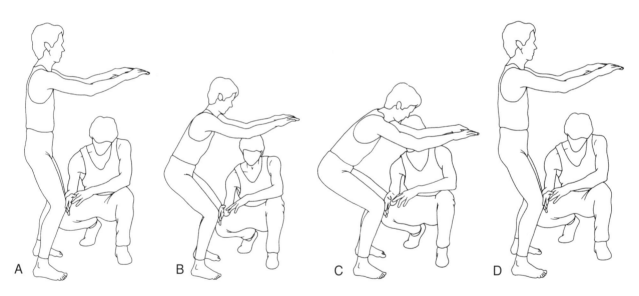

A   B   C   D

Kwa Squat. A) Assume standing posture with both feet parallel (see Figure 9-1, p 154). Partner places forearm and hand on both knees. Partner does not move his or her forearm during the whole exercise. Your knees must continue to touch his or her forearm during the whole exercise, both going up and down. B) Squeeze kwa closed and squat. Spine must remain straight, not arched and arms may be held straight in front of body, with body inclined forward to aid balance. C) Maintain the conditions of A) and B), squeeze kwa and squat lower. If you are stiff or injured, apply the 40 percent or 50 percent rule and recognize that you may never be able to squat as low as shown. D) Maintain the conditions of Figure 9-7A, open kwa and stand up. Make sure your knees do not move.

Figure 9-7

2. Squat from the Kwa

Squat down by gently squeezing your kwa closed, and stand up by expanding or pushing your kwa upward. Under no circumstances should you use your knees to power your squat. There must be a direct line of pressure from your kwa to the arch of your foot, with no weight-bearing pressure exerted on the knee joint, to avoid the possibility of causing injury. The spine must remain straight (without the back muscles being tensed). The spine may incline forward at an angle (as minimal as your body will allow), but your back must not arch. Be sure to keep the perineum open and relax your legs. The squeezing of the kwa is similar to (but not exactly the same as) the way you squeeze to hold in bowel movements.

You may be able to squat only an inch or two in the beginning. People with weak, stiff, or traumatized psoas muscles will be surprised by how little they can squat. This is nothing to worry about. In time, your body may regain the same flexibility seen in a child's ability to squat.

Remember: squat only as low as you can go without the knees moving forward. Squatting to where the buttocks are even with the knees is about the lowest you should want to go. A good practice is to use this kwa squat to pick things up off the floor or from low shelves, or for lifting or putting down heavy objects.

Developing the flexibility of the kwa is essential for neigong, Taoist energy and meditation practices, and the internal martial arts, including tai chi chuan. This simple squatting exercise, which bends and stretches the kwa, is an excellent way to begin stretching the muscles of the kwa and start developing a good elastic quality.

Mette Heinz

Over time, students practicing Cloud Hands learn to connect the energy of the whole body to the spine. The alignments and turning motions of Cloud Hands form the foundation for the movements of tai chi and other internal arts.

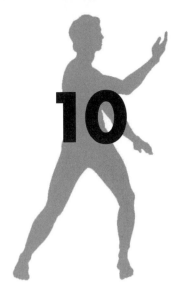

10 Cloud Hands: Spiraling the Upper Body

The Spine Connects the Arms and Legs

A basic function of the Cloud Hands exercise is to connect the energy of your whole body to your spine, which results in the nerves of the spine integrating with the entire body without breaks or dysfunction. This is achieved in three steps.

First, the legs are joined energetically to the pelvis and then to the spine. (You learned how to accomplish this is in Chapter 9). The energy that supports your spine comes from the earth through your legs.

Second, the arms are joined energetically to the spine—you will learn how this is accomplished in this chapter.

Third, the energies from the arms and legs are integrated with each other, through the spine. At this stage, it is very important that the heaven and earth energy connection—from above the head to below the feet—be kept strong during the movements of Cloud Hands.

The arms and legs are essentially the same from the viewpoint of the spine. The hip/shoulder, elbow/knee, and hand/foot have approximately the same vertical and horizontal movements. The coordination between the hands and legs is what allows multidirectional flexibility. Your legs are connected to the earth and your arms to heaven.

Lesson 1   Connecting the Arms to the Spine

This technique involves sinking the shoulders and dropping the elbows.

1. Raise Arms

To begin, raise your arms forward to shoulder height, with the wrists and elbows bent and the hands and fingers parallel to the floor, palms down *(Figure 10-1)*.

The forearms and the upper arms should be parallel to each other; do not let them make a "V" shape, either out or in. Make sure the tips of your elbows point directly to the ground, so that the upper arms, elbows, and forearms are parallel to each other. The object is to have each arm from shoulder to fingers remain on the right and left energy channels of the body *(Figure 10-2A and 10-5)*, which extend from the shoulder's nest down to the kwa on each side.

2. Open the Shoulder Blades

Next, relax your shoulders, letting them drop down, while at the same time rounding the shoulder blades and the back as far as possible. When this movement is done properly, the shoulder blades will seem to disappear.

3. Sink Elbows

Let your elbows drop slightly as if weights were attached to them, pulling them down *(Figure 10-2)*. In order to do this, the area the Chinese call the shoulder's nest *(Figure 10-5)* must be opened, creating a hollow between the inner edge of the

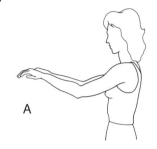

A

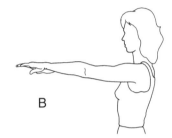

B

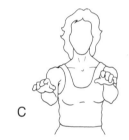

C

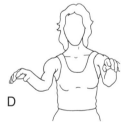

D

Raising Arms to Shoulder Height
A) Correct: Elbows bent.
B) Incorrect: Arms straight.
C) Incorrect: Left arm properly aligned with side channel, but right arm turned out.
D) Incorrect: Left arm slightly turned out, right arm extremely turned out.

Figure 10-1

shoulder and the ribs. This area, in time, becomes extremely soft and very flexible. When this hollow is produced in the shoulder's nest, the shoulders sink and the elbows drop easily and comfortably, without conscious thought.

These steps are all intimately connected, and function primarily to connect the arms energetically to the spine, much like branches grow out of a tree trunk and are not separate from the tree. Most people lack a strong sense of energetic connection between the spine and the arms. Without such connection, the chi from the spine will have difficulty flowing past the shoulders; thus, true energy work will be prevented and the exercise will be limited to muscular activity only.

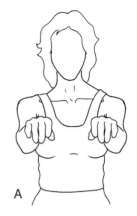

4. Practice the First Exercise Moving with Arms Raised

Close your eyes and continuously shift weight from side to side, as explained in Chapter 9, with your arms in the position indicated in Step 1. You will find that, after a few minutes, your arms probably will have spread out into a "V" shape. Practice this exercise from a few days up to a few weeks, until your arms remain parallel and move only with your body and spine, not independently.

Without practicing this exercise, it is very difficult to get your arms to move in coordination with your spine. The exercise stabilizes the flow of chi from the spine to the arms.

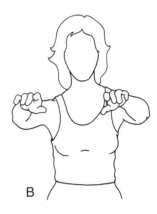

Sinking the Elbows
A) Correct: Elbows tips point down
B) Incorrect: Elbows turned out

Figure 10-2

Two-Person Feedback Exercise

During the practice of this exercise (and some of the others) it is useful to have a partner check to see if you are actually doing what you think you are doing. It is more useful to ask a partner than to look in a mirror. When someone else places you in the correct position, it is possible to compare the way it feels to do an exercise correctly with the way if feels when you think you are doing it correctly. One problem with looking in a mirror is that you are not only doing the exercise, you are also watching, so already there is some dissociation from the feeling in your arms. Second, it is very common to look in a mirror and see only what you want to see. Also, you usually won't have a mirror to practice with, and it is much more important to gain an inner sense of the correct movements and postures. So, if possible, find someone to work with as you practice these exercises.

Lesson 2 Move Elbow Joints to Activate the Spinal Pump

The object of this next exercise is to link the opening and closing of the elbows to the opening and closing of all the tissue from the elbow to the spine (i.e., the upper arm, the shoulder, and shoulder blade). The exercise activates the cerebrospinal pump in the upper spine and neck, which works in association with increasing and decreasing the space between the vertebrae (as the arms extend, the distance increases, and as they bend, it decreases).

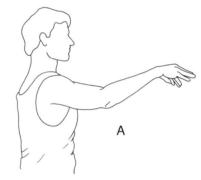

1. Extend Elbows

The procedure is as follows: While keeping the shoulders down, extend the elbows as far forward as possible, so that all the tissue from the spine through the shoulder blades to the shoulder notch is as stretched and open as possible *(Figure 10-3)*.

This extension must not decrease at any point in this exercise—never allow any slack from the elbow to the spine. Your elbow can stay the same distance or extend further away from your spine, but not move closer. The muscles must not become tense or overstretched. Like a rubber band, the muscles from your spine to your fingers must be extended as far as

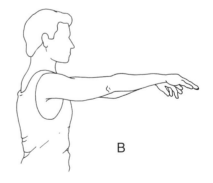

Extending the Elbows. A) Correct: Elbows stretched forward from spine. B) Incorrect: Muscles overstretched and elbows straight.

Figure 10-3

possible so there is no slack in them; yet, also like a rubber band, not so taut that the rubber becomes ready to snap (pull the muscle). Remember the 70 percent rule.

2. Open and Close Elbow Joints to Activate the Spinal Pump

Now bend and straighten the arms to activate the spinal pump and consequent stretching of the vertebrae (remember to only extend and bend to 70 percent of your limit). When you can feel the action of this exercise from the mid-thoracic vertebrae between the shoulder blades (see p. 103 and p. 216), to the top of the neck, you have learned well. This exercise is extremely difficult to learn without the help of a qualified teacher, largely because you have to feel what is going on inside your body at a very subtle level, and usually the instructor has to manipulate the students' arms before they get the exact feeling. While the internal action is extremely powerful, it is almost invisible from the outside, except to the highly trained observer.

Lesson 3 Open the Hip Joint to Turn the Spine

1. Maintain Your Centerline While Turning the Upper and Lower Body

Now we are ready for turning movements, which means it is time to find the centerline of the body. Figure 10-4A shows proper alignment of the body while turning. Note how the centerline is maintained. Figure 10-4B shows how most people turn, breaking the centerline and thereby disengaging the upper body from the lower. With the hands equidistant from the centerline of the body, begin to turn from side to side, remembering all the previously discussed material: lower back straight, hip-knee-ankle connected, back raised, chest rounded, shoulders sunk, elbows dropped, and feet flat. From now on, all new techniques will include all previously learned points.

2. Originate Body Turning from the Kwa

The body has many natural hinges. The joints in your fingers allow the fingers to bend. The wrist joint allows the hand to bend; the elbows allow the arm to

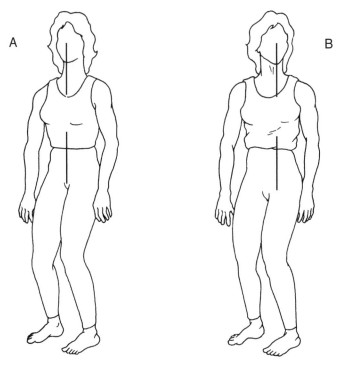

Maintaining the Centerline While Turning the Body
A) Correct: Nose, solar plexus, and groin in one line.
B) Incorrect: Centerline broken.
Figure 10-4

bend. In the hip, this hinge is located in the region around the inguinal groove, which the Chinese call the kwa.

Most people turn to the side by using the muscles between the ribs and hip bone or, even more commonly, by turning their shoulders. From qigong's point of view of body and spinal integrity, this type of turning is incorrect. The body should actually turn from the inguinal groove. Later, when that stabilizes, you can add the muscles of the waist, or *yao* in Chinese. Under no circumstances should you turn the waist using the shoulders, since this breaks the energetic connection between the arms and the spine, and twists the spine.

3. Turn from the Kwa and Keep the Four Points Aligned

In the same way that you do not want to energetically dissociate the arms from the spine, you do not want to dissociate the spine from the hips, waist, and chest. To keep these connected, the movement must originate from the kwa, with the waist

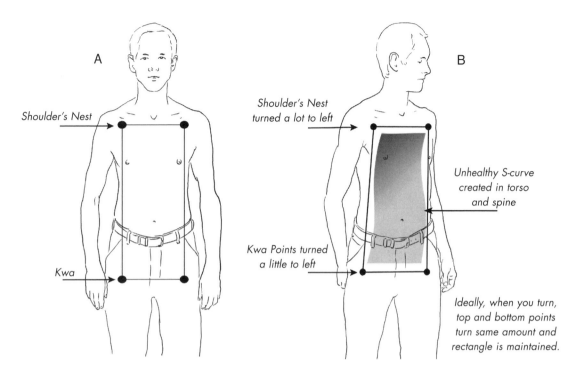

A) Four Points Alignment—Correct: Four Points Maintained as a Rectangle
B) Four Points Alignment—Incorrect: Top Points Turned More than Bottom
Figure 10-5

joining with the hip, and the chest then joining the waist. Practice keeping this connection with the arms held forward as described in Lesson 1. There must be a straight line from the shoulder's nest to the kwa on both sides. These four points must always remain in alignment to prevent the spine from twisting and to cause equal pressure on all the internal organs.

When turning, there is a tendency for the various parts of the body to become disconnected. The legs will need to have their alignment checked, and the arms will again tend to deviate from parallel.

Even if these procedures seem simple, a good teacher is invaluable. You will find there is a great difference between you think you are doing and what you are actually doing. A teacher can be a great help in pointing out discrepancies between the two.

4. The Body Twist Massages the Organs

The primary function of this turning from side to side (other than learning to mesh the trunk, arms, and legs into one unit), is to pressurize the internal organs. Such twisting and wringing of the internal organs will bring them up to optimum condition in the same way that the twisting of a massage practitioner tones your muscles. By keeping the four points aligned, the procedure described here causes chi to accumulate in the internal organs and will connect the spinal energy with the internal organs. This turning also automatically activates the chi flow in the "belt" or collateral acupuncture meridians that wrap around the body.

5. Shift Weight from One Leg to the Other

In this exercise, the weight shifts completely from leg to leg as the waist simultaneously turns from side to side. In the middle position, the weight is evenly distributed on both feet and the waist is facing forward. Move the weight 100 percent to the left leg and turn the waist to the left. Move back through the middle position, and then turn to the right until your weight is 100 percent on the right leg. Repeat. Many people will unconsciously tend to do the opposite: when turning to the right, they will keep their weight on the left leg. Beginners will initially find it easier to shift 100 percent onto one leg before turning. Over time, however, weight shifting and waist turning should happen simultaneously.

Lesson 4 Sink One Side to Raise the Other

The next technique establishes a simple pumping action in the body, so that energy rises up one side of the body and drops down the other.

1. Sink One Hand, Feel the Other Hand Rise

Begin with one arm raised to shoulder level and the other at the side with palm facing toward the ground. As you lower one hand, the other simultaneously rises. The arm sinking downwards should create a feeling of energy or blood descending down the corresponding leg and into the floor. The sinking of energy down one side of the body should be felt to simultaneously cause energy to rise up the other side and lift the opposite hand up. As you practice this pulley action, it is imperative that the sinking hand causes the other hand to rise, and not the other way around. Energy sinking down the body will always cause energy to rise, while raising energy up the body may or may not cause energy to sink.

2. Coordinate Sinking the Arm and Leg on the Same Side

Next, shift the weight from side to side so that the leg receiving the weight is on the same side as the sinking hand—when the left hand is sinking the left leg is gaining weight, and vice versa. This will cause energy to rise up the opposite extending arm and leg.

Lesson 5 "Spinning Silk" with the Arms and Legs

1. Spiraling Energy that Gives Natural Power

When done correctly, Cloud Hands involves the spiraling of the arms. Natural joint movement and energy flow in human beings moves in spirals, similar to the structure of the DNA helix. Most people only use this spiraling action minimally, athletes use it more, and people with exceptional physical and movement abilities, who are able to keep these abilities into old age, use this spiraling action almost exclusively.

In tai chi chuan, this action is called twisting silk or *chan sz jin*, which is a metaphor for the way silk is spiraled out of the silk cocoon so that the threads do not break. In hsing-i and bagua, this same idea is called *luo shuen jin*—or drilling or twisting strength, which is taken from the action of drilling a screw. The twisting of the muscles, which follows the natural spiraling energy in the body, can be first observed in babies. The first attempts of babies at moving their arms and legs, and turning over and crawling, is done with spiraling movements, not straight-line muscular movement.

2. Practice Spiraling with the Entire Arm

To learn to be aware of this spiraling energy, it is best to first concentrate on the arms, and later add the waist and legs. Place your hands to the side, by your hips, with your fingers pointing straight ahead. The wrists are bent so the palms and tips of the elbows face the floor and press slightly downwards. Beginning with the least coordinated arm, slowly and smoothly raise and turn the hand, until it is at a

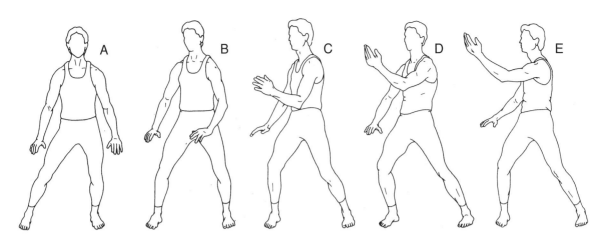

The Cloud Hands Movement is a Continuous Flow.
The positions shown are transitional guides, not static end points.
A) Starting posture: Weight 100 percent on left leg, arms at sides.
B), C), D) & E) Shift weight to 100 percent on right leg, as the body turns to the right.
Simultaneously, spiral and raise the left arm.

Figure 10-6A-E

height somewhere between the chest and nose. The higher your hand goes, the greater the stretch of your back and shoulder blades. Remember the 70 percent rule, and only increase the height of your hands as your back opens up. The hand ends on the centerline, with the palm facing upwards and toward the face with the forearm at a 45° rounded angle. The arm then returns along the same circular path, ending in its original position.

As in all Taoist body practices, the spiraling of the arm begins at the space between the spine and shoulder blade, continues through the shoulder, upper arm, elbow, and forearm, and completes in the fingers.

The trick is to turn the hand exactly in proportion to the rate that the hand is rising or sinking, so that when the hand has risen 10 percent of the distance from the hip to nose it has rotated 10 percent. At the midpoint from hip to nose, the palms would be facing each other or 50 percent rotated, and so on.

During this procedure, it is extremely important that the armpits are open and the arms and ribs do not touch. For women, it is very important to maintain, at all times, at least a distance the size of a fist between the breasts and the arms, especially the sides of the arms. Also, the elbow is always bent and sinking

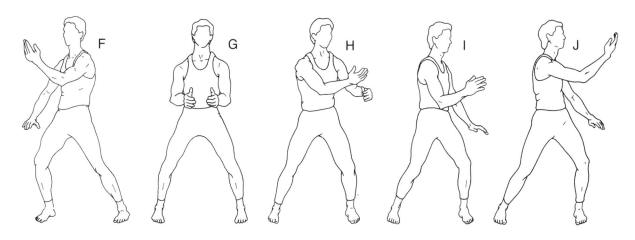

F) Begin to shift and turn to the left. Simultaneously, the upper arm begins to spiral
and sink, the lower arm begins to spiral and rise.
G) Mid-point: Weight equally distributed on both legs, body faces straight ahead,
palms face each other on opposite sides of the centerline.
H), I) & J) Continue to shift and turn until weight is 100 percent on left leg, body turned to left.
Simultaneously, spiral the arms until the left hand is palm down at side of
hip and right hand is opposite the nose.

Figure 10-6F-J

downwards, so that at all times there would be room for an egg or small orange
to fit in the crook of the elbow. The shoulders stay down while the arms rise.

3. Coordinate the Arm Spiral with the Turn in the Kwa

The rising, falling, and spiraling of the arm is then joined with turning from the hip
and shifting the weight. As the waist turns, the arm rounds and makes an arc to
accommodate the turning of the waist. The thumb finishes at approximately groin
height facing the hip bone on the centerline of the side of the body, and the fingers
point in the same direction as the groin. In fact, the groin, solar plexus, nose
(head) and fingers, as well as the four points of the kwa and shoulder's nest, *point
in the same direction at all times*. The side with the palm pointing down is the side
with the weight. Repeat the same procedure with the opposite hand and arm.

4. Twist the Leg Muscles

The thigh and calf muscles should twist in the same direction as the waist is turning,
and at a speed proportional to that of the arm twist. The twisting, or
wrapping, of the leg muscles has two functions. First, it prevents damage to the
knee joint. Second, it spirals the tissue of the leg. This will prepare you for more

advanced practices, which teach you to spiral energy through the body. More
information about this is discussed in Chapter 15.

5. Practice the Complete Cloud Hands Movement

This step requires both hands to work simultaneously, which coordinates the left
and right sides of the brain.

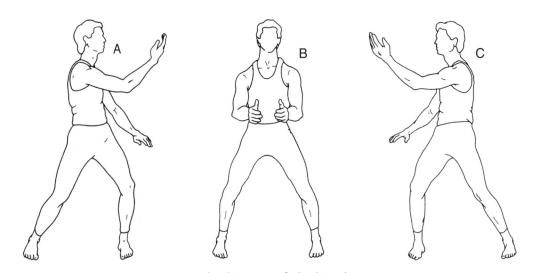

Landmark Positions of Cloud Hands
A) Start with your weight completely on the left leg. B) Weight 50/50, facing straight ahead, in the middle of
the transition between the weight being 100 percent on the right or left leg. C) When you turn to the right,
weight is completely on your right leg.

Figure 10-7

Start with your weight completely on the left leg and your body turned to the left
(Figure 10-7A). Your left hand will be palm down by the left hip and the right hand
will be palm up in front of your nose.

Slowly begin to shift your weight to the right. When you reach the midpoint,
your weight will be 50/50 and you will be facing straight ahead *(Figure 10-7B)*.
Both of your hands will be at the same height, palms facing each other, near
the centerline of the body. When you finish turning to the right, the left hand will
be palm up at your nose and your right hand will be palm down at the side of
your hip, aligned with the armpit. Both hands will be rotating at a speed exactly
proportional to the speed that they are rising and falling. With practice, Cloud

Hands should become one smooth movement, rather than two separate movements on each side.

At the end of shifting the weight to either leg, it is best not to come to a complete stop and remain there in a static position, even for only a brief moment. Ideally, at the end of either movement, shown in Figure 10-7A or C, let your hands continue to make small circular movements, so that the flow of the hands reversing their rising and falling positions remains continuous and fluid, without jerky stops and starts. The weight shifting from one leg to the other should also be equally smooth and continuous.

Though Cloud Hands can be fairly difficult, this exercise can also give the body a greater sense of freedom and energy than it has ever known before.

6. Power the Movement of the Arms by the Turning of the Hips

In Cloud Hands and the three swings that follow, the movement of the arms must be powered by the turnings of the hips, which over time increases the movement of chi in the entire body. The more completely energy flows between the legs, torso and spine, the easier it is to have chi flow through the arms, making them go higher. The purpose of Cloud Hands and the swings is to get energy moving strongly in the middle of the body: until then it will not be fully able to express itself at the extremities of the arms and legs.

Once you learn the mechanics of the three swings that follow, to reap their full benefits, do not force the arms to move higher. Instead let the arms relax and move or swing away from and toward the body on their own accord. At first, the arms will not go very high. It may take months for the arms to rise as high as your belly button and even more time to get the arms as high as your solar plexus.

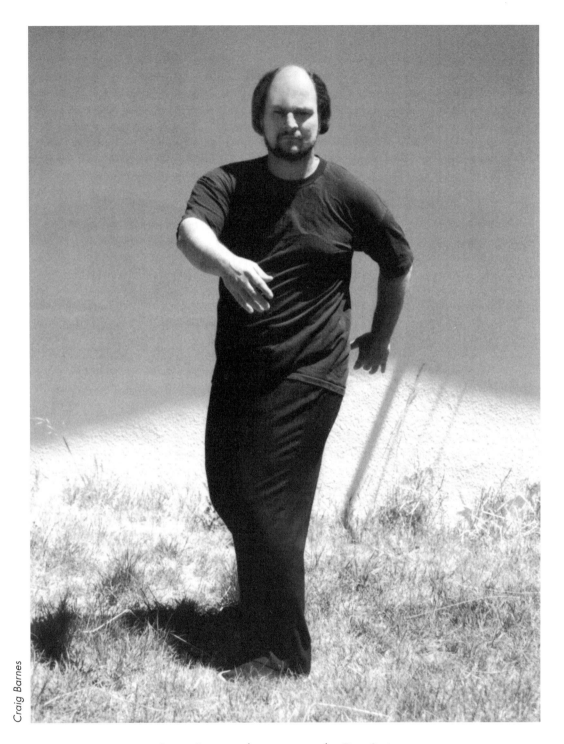

Craig Barnes

Bruce Frantzis demonstrates the First Swing.

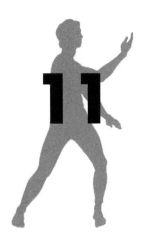

11 The First Swing

The Swings Energize Vital Organs and Joints

The next three exercises, called *swai shou* in Chinese, and generally referred to as "the swings" in English, have the basic function of energizing the upper, lower, and middle internal organs, as well as fully opening up the joints of the hips, shoulders, elbows and hands.

The Three Tantiens and Jiao of Chinese Medicine

From the point of view of practicing chi development, there are three main tantiens, each of which has a different function. An illustration of the three tantiens is shown on p. 239.

The lower tantien, near the belly, is the source of life in the physical body. The middle tantien, located around the center of the sternum (i.e., the heart) is the energy center through which a person connects and forms relationships with other living things and their emotions, as well as being the source of thoughts and intentions. This is the source of compassion and benevolence, as well as the place where negative emotions are transformed.

The upper tantien, located at the third eye, is responsible for connections with time, space, noncorporeal beings, subtle forms of thought, and other dimensions and places.

Beginning qigong is primarily concerned with the lower tantien. More advanced qigong and Taoist meditation focuses on the two higher tantiens.

The three swings involve the three burners, or *jiao*, of the body. The lower jiao, which begins below the lower tantien and extends down to the floor, is primarily concerned with the functioning of the legs, urinogenital health, the large intestine and the kidneys (which are also influenced by the middle burner).

The middle jiao extends from the tantien to the solar plexus and is responsible for the health of most of the organs—the small intestine, spleen, pancreas, liver, stomach, and gallbladder. The upper jiao extends from the chest to the top of the head, including the arms. It is responsible for the health of the heart, lungs, brain, and arms.

Each of the three swings energizes one particular burner. The First Swing has the primary function of opening the chi of the lower internal organs, the urinogenital area, the stomach, and the intestines. This swing will be of particular interest to people with constipation, sexual weakness, and kidney difficulties—both in terms of Western and Chinese medicine—and is particularly helpful for those who have cold and clammy hands and feet.

Lesson 1 Leg and Hip Movement Is the Same as Cloud Hands

1. Turn from the Kwa and Shift Weight

The shifting of the weight, the opening and closing of the joints of the legs, the turning of the waist and the bending at the inguinal cut (kwa) are essentially the same as you learned in Cloud Hands (see Chapter 10).

2. Increase Speed of Twisting

Now, however, the weight is shifted from leg to leg fairly quickly. Begin practicing the movement faster than slow motion and yet not as quickly as possible. It is extremely important that the head remain on the centerline of your body, along with the nose, the breastbone, the navel, and the groin, and that the four points of the shoulder's nest and kwa stay aligned *(Figure 11-1A).*

3. Keep the Proper Hip-Knee-Ankle Alignment

Although the leg and hip movements are essentially the same as in Cloud Hands, it is worth re-emphasizing that the perineum must stay open, the body must turn by folding at the inguinal groove, the knees must be slightly bent (especially easy to forget with the weightless leg), the ankles and knees must be properly aligned, and the thigh muscles must twist in the same direction as the waist so that no strain is created in the lower back or the knees.

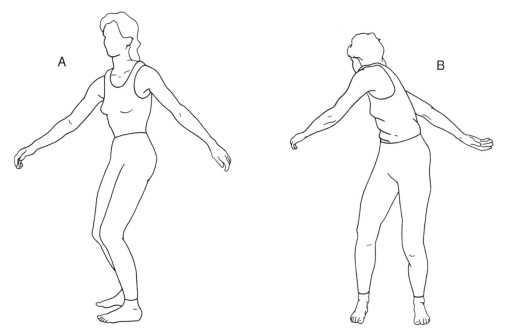

Maintaining integrity of centerline. A) Correct: Nose, solar plexus and groin in a line.
B) Incorrect: Shoulders and head turned more than hips.

Figure 11-1

Central Energy Channel

According to Taoist tradition, the central channel or core energy channel is the most important energetic pathway in the body (see p. 239). This line of energy runs vertically directly through the center of the body. A cut directly down the central axis of the body would bisect this energy core, which goes from the center of the head right down through the perineum, and continues through the center of the bone marrow of the arms and legs. This central vertical core of energy is the original energetic source of the formation of the human body from conception onward, manifesting in the development of the spine, the arms, and the legs, according to Taoist qigong tradition. As you turn your body, you should keep your attention on your core channel and use it as the axis of your turn. However, you should also focus part of your attention on your lower tantien, which is on this core channel, so that it is also the center of your turn. It is important that you move and turn equally from both places as this results in the largest output of energy to all the systems of the body. This point also applies to Cloud Hands, but it is easier to learn to move from both places evenly here, in the swings, and then go back and include it in Cloud Hands.

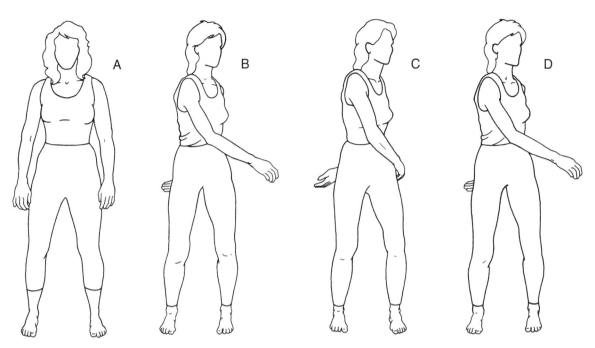

The First Swing. This movement is a continuous flow. The positions shown are transitional guides, not static end points. A) Starting posture: Weight equally distributed on both legs, body facing straight ahead, arms at sides. B) & C) Shift weight 100 percent to left leg and simultaneously turn to left; hands will swing in to touch body.

Figure 11-2A-D

Lesson 2 Arm Movements

1. Coordinate Arm Movements with Turns

Face forward with your feet parallel and your hands at your sides *(Figure 11-2A)*. As you begin to shift weight and turn to the left, your hands begin swinging out *(Figure 11-2B)*. As you finish the weight shift, the left arm will lightly touch the back of the upper hip with the back of the hand and the right arm will lightly touch the front of the belly or thigh with the palm of your hand *(Figure 11-2C)*.

As you begin to turn back to the center, the hands will begin to swing out *(Figure 11-2D)*. As your weight shifts 50/50 to both feet and the body faces center, the hands will swing out to their maximum distance from the body *(Figure 11-2E)*. As you begin to turn to the right, the hands will begin to swing in *(Figure 11-2F)*. As you complete the weight shift and turn, the right arm will lightly touch the back of the thigh with the back of the hand and the left arm will lightly touch the front of the belly, hip or thigh with the palm of the hand *(Figure 11-2G)*.

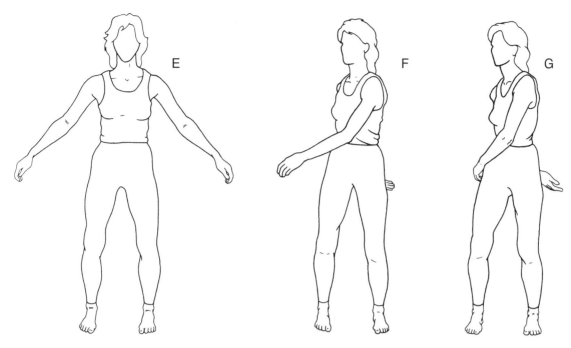

D) & E) Begin to shift weight to the right and simultaneously turn back to mid-point; hands will swing out.
F) & G) Shift weight 100 percent to the right and simultaneously turn to right; hands will swing in to touch body.

Figure 11-2E-G

2. The Swinging Arms Must Be Totally Limp

The arms dangle from the shoulders, without using muscular control to move them in any direction. In other words, they should hang as though they were limp. Then use your awareness to make the shoulders, elbows, wrists, palms, and fingers as soft and relaxed as possible. With each swing, as the internal organs get warmed up, try to make the arms softer and softer until the joints of the arm feel as though they are filled with water or a soft warm liquid.

3. Power the Swing with Centrifugal Force

During the course of these swings, the arms will never act independently. They will simply passively be moved by the centrifugal force of the body as it swings to the left and right. Turning from the hips generates the force that moves the arms. A turn to the right side will bend the left arm toward the front of the body and the right arm toward the back of the body *(Figure 11-3)*. A turn to the left will do just the opposite.

As the centrifugal force swings the arms away from the body, the joints of the arms and shoulder should naturally open without you deliberately moving them. As the centrifugal force swings the arms toward the body, the joints of the arms and shoulders bend and close. All these actions must be accomplished by internal feeling, not looking. There is a great difference between intellectually knowing what your left and right sides are doing and kinesthetically sensing what your left and right sides are doing. Again, it is preferable to work with a partner who will help you by touching your body to give you accurate feedback. Relying on a mirror will provide only a visual/intellectual understanding.

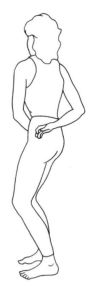

It is of the utmost importance to begin to use awareness to relax and allow the elbow joint to let go. Under no circumstances should you independently move your arm muscles or bend the hands and arms. Continuously sink your chi. The shoulders should stay totally sunken and relaxed.

Turning to right propels right arm to back of body, left arm to front.

Figure 11-3

4. Hands Lightly Tap Kidneys and Abdomen

In the beginning, your arms will probably not bend higher than the top of your thighs at the end of your turn to the side. As relaxation of the arms and elbow joints increases and your chi sinks more, the arms will offer less and less resistance to the centrifugal force being generated by the turning of the waist.

As this occurs, and as the turning of the waist becomes more and more fluid, the bend in the arms at the elbows will increase, until the forearms are eventually parallel to the floor. At this point, the hands will be lightly tapping the abdomen from the front and the kidneys from the back. Be gentle around the kidney area and tap it only with minimal force. Hitting the kidneys with excessive force is a sure way to hurt yourself, possibly even fatally. Kidney blows have been outlawed from boxing due to their danger. Although there are qigong techniques for learning to absorb kidney punches, such techniques require the continued guidance of a master.

During the swings, it is extremely important that the space underneath the armpits stays open and the arms do not touch the ribs.

In time, with proficiency, as the arms come inwards they will bring healthy chi into the body, and as they swing away they will release stale or useless chi—in much the same way that oxygen is inhaled and carbon dioxide exhaled.

5. Do Not Drop Your Head

One of the most common mistakes made, which usually proves to be transitional, is that, as the practitioner relaxes the arms and waist more and more, the head drops down. For most people, the more they relax, the more the head tends to fall forward. This is a basic neurological reflex; as people go into a kinesthetic mode (i.e., feeling the body), the underlying tendency is for the eyes and head to drop and spine to sag. During these exercises, it is very important to be aware of this tendency and correct it (i.e., keep your head straight up and jaw parallel to the ground), so that the body is relaxed internally but does not collapse (see p.xxx).

6. Keep Hands Soft

In this swing, the arms and only the arms should collapse like a wet noodle, which brings us to the last detail: The hands must become totally soft, like a baby's. Avoid locking the fingers in any position, and keep the palms of the hands very soft and pliable. The amount of tension held in the hands indicates and affects the tension that is held in the rest of the body. Relaxing the hands will gradually spread relaxation throughout your whole nervous system.

Two-Person Exercise to Release Shoulder and Elbow Tension

Particular attention must be paid to relaxing the elbow joints and removing any strength from them. To learn what it is like to have no strength in the arms, have someone hold your upper arm parallel to the floor, with the elbow bent so that the forearm points to the sky. Relax the arm completely. The holder then lets go of the forearm, which should, if the elbow is relaxed, drop with the force of gravity. The habitual tension that most people carry in their arms usually does not let the arm drop immediately but only after a slight lag time. Practice this a few times until the arm falls down easily and comfortably, as a result of the release of all control and strength in the arm.

Next, raise the whole arm straight up above your head and then let go. Repeat this until the whole arm can fall toward the floor in a relaxed manner, without any muscular contractions causing it to get stuck on the way down. Relaxation, increased circulation, smooth nerve flow down the arm, and an increase in chi will gradually allow the movements of this exercise to become smoother and smoother.

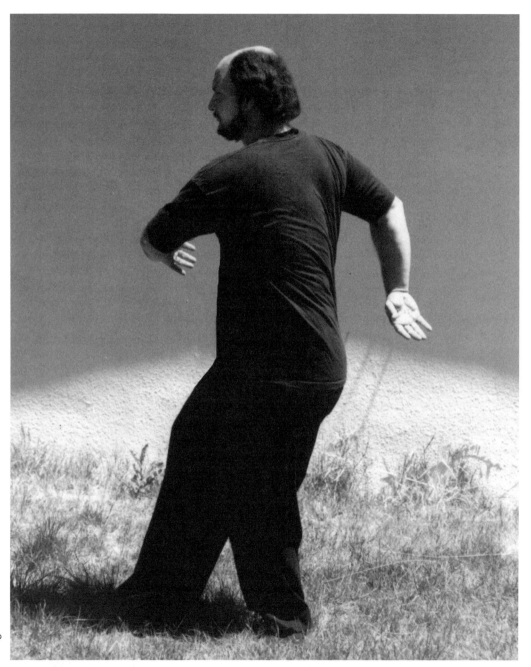

Craig Barnes

Bruce Frantzis demonstrates the Second Swing.

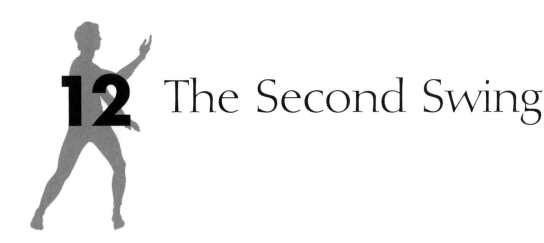

12 The Second Swing

The Second Swing Strengthens the Liver and Spleen and Dissolves Stress

The purpose of the Second Swing is to energize and strengthen the middle internal organs, including the spleen, liver, stomach, and pancreas, and the glands such as the adrenals. The footwork is essentially the same for the Second and Third Swings, though different from the footwork of the First Swing. The arm movements of the First and Second Swing are essentially the same.

The Challenge: Shift Weight and Turn at the Kwa

The basis of all correct movement in tai chi chuan, as well as in hsing-i and bagua, involves physically and energetically joining the leg and waist together as the body shifts weight. This applies to any turning or stepping movements and any turns and dodges from side to side. The difficulty lies in getting the legs and waist to turn through sinking into, and expanding from, the inguinal cut (kwa), and not by twisting from the knee, which can slowly damage the lower back and leg joints. Learning the correct weight shifting and turning techniques whether for health or power generation, is central to all Taoist internal martial arts movements–or as it is more poetically put in *The Tai Chi Classics*, "If there is an error, look to the waist and the legs."

Lesson 1 Hip and Leg Movements

1. Shift Weight to Right Leg 100 Percent, While Facing Forward

A) Begin with your weight equally distributed on both legs, arms at your side and head and feet facing forward *(Figure 12-1)*.

B) While still facing forward, shift your weight 100 percent to your right leg (not shown). Caution: If the weight is only shifted 50 percent when going to the side this can easily lead to knee strain. All weight shifts must be 100 percent.

C) By the time you finish your weight shift, lift up the left heel so that only the ball of the left foot is touching the ground, (this is not visible in Figure 12-1). The foot, knee joint, crest of the pubic bone, four points of the shoulder's nest and kwa, and the groin should all point in the same direction, that is, straight ahead. The feet should be parallel.)

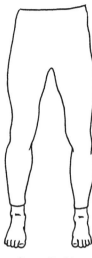

Center Position

Figure 12-1

2. Pivot The Body to the Left: Left Hip, Leg and Foot Move as One Unit

A) Place both hands on the belly. For the remainder of Lesson 1, your hands will remain there. It is easier to focus on turning properly if you do not have to think about the placement of the hands.

B) Before you start turning, make sure that the weight is 100 percent on the right leg.

C) With the weight fully on the right leg, pivot your body to the left. Keep your right leg still and pivot from your right kwa and hip joint. Let the unweighted left hip, leg and foot be swung as a unit in an arc, following the pivot of the right hip. Let the ball of the left foot slide along the ground. Let the left leg and foot be moved to the same degree that the right hip pivots *(Figure 12-2A and B)*. If the right hip pivots 45 degrees, the left leg, heel and toes will also move 45 degrees.

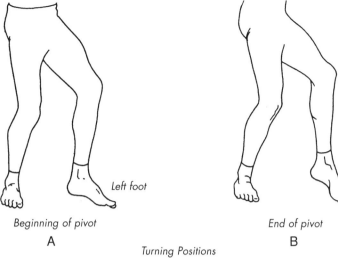

Beginning of pivot
A

Turning Positions

End of pivot
B

Figure 12-2

D) During the turn and especially at the end of the turn, these parts of your body should all be facing/pointing in the same direction:

- Centerline of your torso where your nose, solar plexus, navel and groin are all aligned in a straight line.
- Centerline of your unweighted foot, which is located along the midline between your middle toe, ball of the foot and the center of your heel.
- Crest of your hip.
- Four points of the torso (the kwa and shoulder's nest on each side).

E) During the turn, the weighted right leg neither bends nor straightens further.

F) Do not move or twist the knee of your weighted leg as you pivot. It is important that the pivoting comes from the hips, and not from any twisting of the knee. As you pivot relax your weighted leg thigh muscles, letting them move in the same direction as the hips. This will prevent the torque created by the hips from pulling or twisting the weighted leg knee in any direction

G) Pivot to the left only as far as 70 percent of your capacity. Doing so will make it much easier to keep the alignments of D.

3. Pivot on the Right Hip Back to Center

A) Again, let the unweighted left hip, leg and foot follow the movement of the right hip back to center. The leg itself does not initiate the pivot *(Figure 12-3A)*.

B) When you have completed the pivot back to center, put your left heel down and shift your weight so that it is again distributed evenly on both feet. Your torso is facing forward and your feet are parallel *(Figure 12-3B)*.

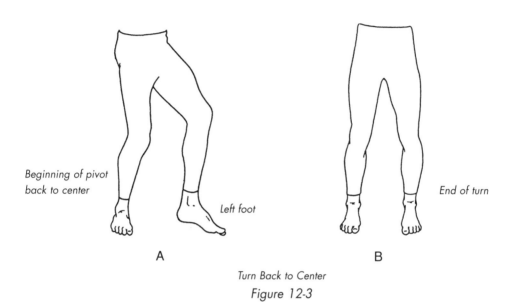

Beginning of pivot back to center

Left foot

End of turn

A

B

Turn Back to Center

Figure 12-3

C). Do not allow the feet to splay. They must remain parallel when you return to center *(Figure 12-4A)*.

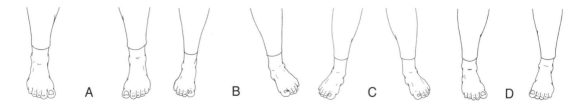

A   B   C   D

A) Correct: Feet parallel. B) Incorrect: One foot splayed outward.
C) Incorrect: Both feet splayed outward. D) Incorrect: Feet turned inward.

Figure 12–4

4. Shift Weight to Left Leg 100 Percent, While Facing Forward

A) While still facing forward, shift your weight 100 percent to your left leg (not visible in Figure 12-5).

B) Lift up the right heel so that only the ball of the right foot is touching the ground (not shown in illustration). Maintain the alignments of Step 2D.

5. Pivot The Body to the Right: Right Hip, Leg and Foot Move as One Unit

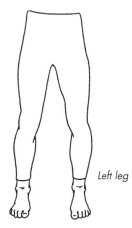

Left leg

Figure 12-5

A) With weight fully on the left leg, pivot your body to the right *(Figure 12-6A and B)*. Keep your left leg still and pivot from your left kwa and hip joint. Let the right hip, leg and foot be swung as a unit in an arc, following the pivot of the left hip. Let the ball of the right foot slide along the ground. Let the right leg and foot be moved to the same degree that the left hip pivots. If the left hip pivots 45 degrees, the right leg, heel and toes will also move 45 degrees.

B) As you pivot, maintain the alignments described in 2D.

C) The left leg neither straightens nor bends further.

D) Pivot the body to the right only as far as 70 percent of your capacity.

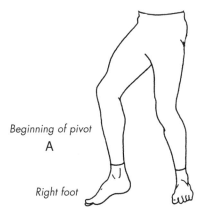

Beginning of pivot

A

Right foot

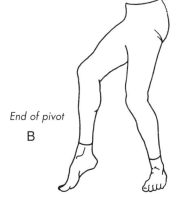

End of pivot

B

Figure 12-6

6. Pivot on the Left Hip Back to Center

A) Again, let the right hip, leg and foot follow the movement of the left hip back to center. The leg does not initiate the turn *(Figure 12-7A)*.

B) When you have completed the pivot back to center *(Figure 12-7B)*, put your right heel down and shift your weight so that it is again distributed evenly on both feet. Your torso is facing forward and your feet are parallel.

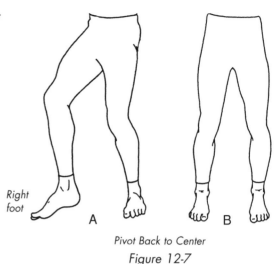

Right foot

A   B

Pivot Back to Center

Figure 12-7

7. Repeat Steps 1-6

This lesson should be done in practice segments of 5 minutes at a time. Your goal is to have the leg of the unweighted foot follow the pivoting of the hip of the weighted leg. This could take many weeks or more. Do not attempt Lesson 2 till the turns are smooth and comfortable.

Important Points to Remember

1. Weight must shift 100 percent to each leg before the pivot is initiated.
2. Do not turn your knees as you pivot your hips to either side.
3. The unweighted hip, leg and foot follows the pivot of the hips.
4. When you pivot back to the center, your feet must be parallel before you shift weight to the other foot. Do not allow the feet to splay.

Lesson 2 Lift and Lower the Foot

In this lesson, the turning is essentially the same as Lesson 1, with this variant. You will be picking up the unweighted foot slightly off the ground; lightly touching the ground with the ball of the foot when you have completed a turn to the right or left; and picking up the foot again, when you turn back to center. This technique is ideally done in all the leg movements of the second and third swing. In this lesson, only the illustrations for major postures are shown, not the transitions. These are shown in Lesson 1 and in Figure 12-14.

This exercise provides two distinct benefits: 1) It circulates significantly more chi in your internal organs and between your spine and legs; 2) It much more strongly joins, aligns and connects the legs to the hips, abdomen and spine.

1. Shift Weight to Right Leg 100 Percent, While Facing Forward

A) Place both hands on the belly. For the remainder of Lesson 2, your hands will remain there.

B) Begin with your weight equally distributed on both legs, arms at your side and head and feet facing forward *(Figure 12-8)*.

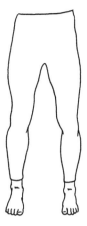

Figure 12-8

C) While still facing forward, shift your weight 100 percent to your right leg (not shown in illustration).

D) At the very end of your weight shift, as you begin to transit into the turn, lift up the left foot an inch or two off the ground (not shown in illustration).

2. Pivot the Body to the Left: Hip, Leg and Foot Move as One Unit

A) With the weight still on the right leg, and the left foot off the ground, pivot to the left. Let the left leg and foot be swung in an arc to the same degree that the right hip pivots. As you pivot, maintain the alignments of Lesson 1, 2D.

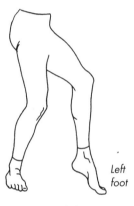

Left foot

Figure 12-9

B) Pivot to the left only as far as 70 percent of your capacity. When you reach the endpoint of the pivot to the left, lower your leg and lightly touch the ground with the ball of the left foot *(Figure 12-9)*.

3. Pivot the Right Hip Back to Center

A) When you begin to pivot back to center, again lift the left foot slightly off the ground (not shown). As you pivot, let the left hip, leg and foot follow the movement of the hip back to center. Maintain the alignments of Lesson 1, 2D.

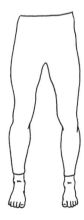

Figure 12-10

B) When you have completed the pivot back to center, put the ball of your left foot down and then almost instantly the heel and shift your weight so that it is again distributed evenly on both feet. Your torso is facing forward and your feet are parallel *(Figure 12-11)*.

4. Shift Weight to Left Leg 100 Percent, While Facing Forward

A) While still facing forward, shift your weight 100 percent to your left leg (not shown in illustration).

B) Lift up the right foot an inch or two off the ground, to transit into the turn, (not shown in illustration).

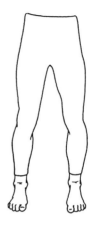

Figure 12-11

5. Pivot The Body to the Right: Hip, Leg and Foot Move as One Unit

A) With the weight still on the left leg, and the right foot lifted off the ground, pivot to the right (not shown in illustration). Let the right leg and foot be swung in an arc to the same degree that the left hip pivots.

B) Pivot to the right only as far as 70 percent of your capacity. When you reach the endpoint of the pivot to the right lightly touch the ground with the ball of the right foot *(Figure 12-12)*.

Right foot

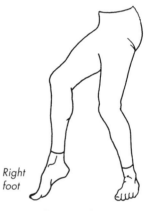

Figure 12-12

6. Pivot on the Left Hip Back to Center

A) As you begin to pivot back to center, lift the right foot slightly off the ground. Again, let the right leg follow the movement of the hip back to center.

B) When you have completed the pivot back to center. put your right foot on the ground and shift your weight so that it is again distributed evenly on both feet. Your torso is facing forward and your feet are parallel *(Figure 12-13)*.

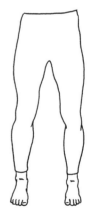

Figure 12-13

7. Repeat Steps 1-6.

This lesson should be done in practice segments of 5 minutes at a time. Your goal is to have the leg of the unweighted foot follow the pivoting of the hip of the weighted leg. Do not attempt Lesson 3 until the turns are smooth and comfortable.

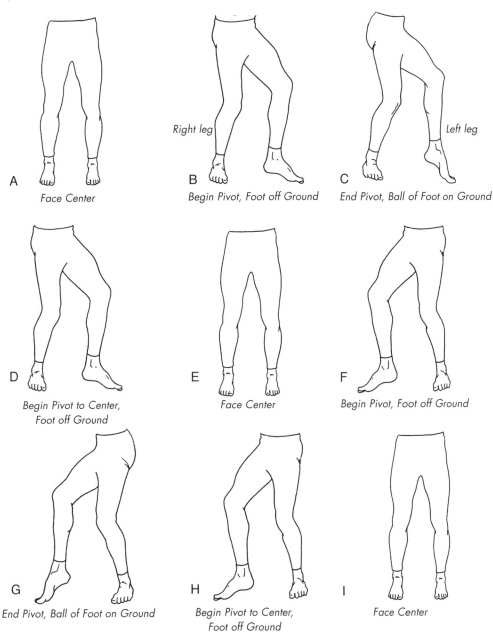

A Face Center

B *Right leg* Begin Pivot, Foot off Ground

C *Left leg* End Pivot, Ball of Foot on Ground

D Begin Pivot to Center, Foot off Ground

E Face Center

F Begin Pivot, Foot off Ground

G End Pivot, Ball of Foot on Ground

H Begin Pivot to Center, Foot off Ground

I Face Center

Complete Leg Movements of Second Swing with Transitions
Figure 12-14

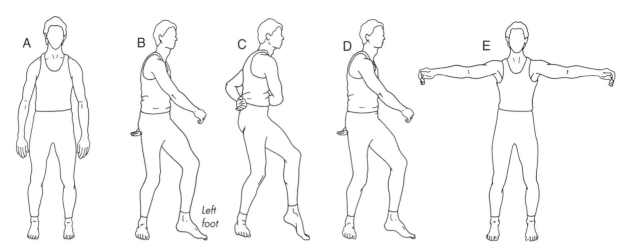

The Second Swing. This movement is a continuous flow. Postures shown are transitional guides, not static end points.
A) Starting posture: Weight equally distributed on both legs, body faces straight ahead, arms at sides.
B) Shift weight 100 percent to right leg, begin pivot to left (allowing left leg to swing in an arc); arms swing out.
C) Continue to pivot to left (set down ball of left foot); arms will swing in to touch the body.
D) Begin to pivot back to the center; arms will swing out.
E) Mid-point: Weight equally distributed on two legs, body faces straight ahead; arms are at apex of extension.

Figure 12-15A-E

Lesson 3 The Arm Movements for the Second Swing

1. The Arm Motions of the Second Swing Are the Same as the First Swing, Except the Hands Go Up Higher

The mechanics of the arm movements for the Second Swing are the same as those for the First Swing: As you turn, the arms swing out *(Figures 12-15B, D, E, H and I)*. As you finish the turn, one palm touches the front of the body and the back of the other hand touches the back of the body *(Figures 12-15C and G)*.

As your hips loosen and the arc of the hips increases, your hands will eventually swing higher, eventually hitting your torso between the navel and the solar plexus, where the middle internal organs are located.

Remember to power the arm movements from the rotation of the hips and body (see chapter 11, p. 185). Do not force the arms to swing.

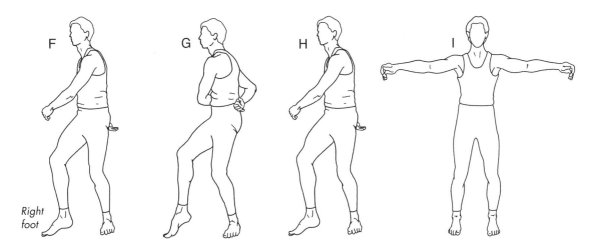

F) Shift weight 100 percent to left leg, begin pivot to right (allowing right leg to swing in an arc); arms will swing in.

G) Continue to pivot to right (set down ball of right foot); arms will swing in to touch body.

H) Begin to pivot back to the center; arms will swing out.

I) Mid-point: Weight equally distributed on two legs, body faces straight ahead; arms are at apex of extension. The Second Swing now continuously repeats starting from 12-15B (with the arms swinging in) to 12-15I.

Figure 12-15F-I

2. Let Chi from Palms Penetrate to the Vital Organs

Touch the body very lightly in the beginning and, over time, let your hands slowly tap the body harder, allowing the energy to penetrate farther and farther inside. At the beginning, the sensation from the hands will only be superficial, but eventually it will penetrate deeply inside the body.

Under no circumstances hit the body with any force or penetration in a spot where there is pain due to a malfunctioning internal organ or injury, and always tap the kidney area gently. If there is pain, touch the area as lightly as possible or even stop the hands just short of touching. (See section regarding kidney blows on p. 186.)

3. Spiraling Arms Circulate Chi

As the arms swing away from the body, let the muscles and connective tissues of the arms naturally twist outward away from the torso so that the energy goes from the tantien up the spine, to the fingertips, and out into space away from the body. As the arms come in, energy from the air enters the body through the hands as your arms twist inward towards your torso. This is another form of energy circulation, from center to periphery and from periphery to center. Now add this spiraling arm movement to the way you practice the First Swing in Chapter 11.

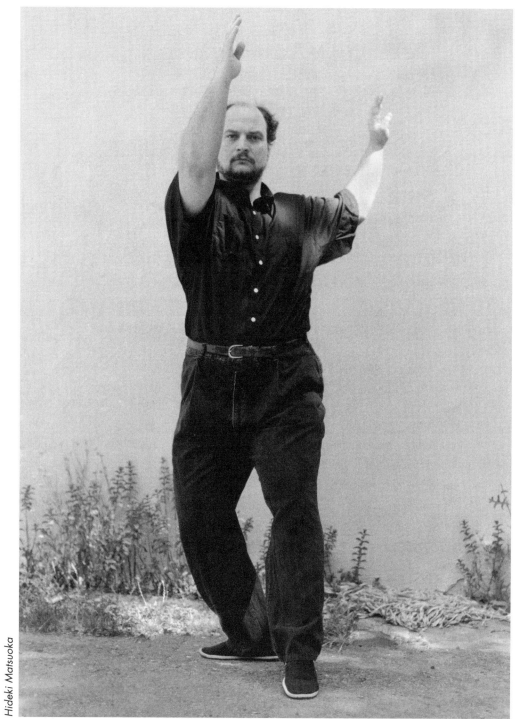

Hideki Matsuoka

Bruce Frantzis demonstrates the Third Swing.

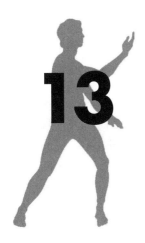

13 The Third Swing

The Third Swing Invigorates Chi in the Upper Body

The Third Swing has a number of functions. Most importantly, it works the upper internal organs (the heart and lungs) and energizes the brain. Secondly, it adds spring to the vertebrae, so that they open and close with greater ease. Thirdly, it begins to open up the rotation of the shoulder joint, as well as the vertebrae of the neck, which are directly associated with the movement of the shoulders. Fourthly, it completely opens the hips and the kwa. Finally, the Third Swing teaches the body to instantaneously relax and let go on command. Once an understanding of the body's energy has been gained through these qigong exercises, it is possible to use the mind to direct the body so that movement is natural and effortless, not forced.

Lesson 1 Leg and Kwa Movements

The footwork of the Third Swing is essentially the same as for the Second Swing, including picking up and touching the ground with the unweighted foot. Unlike the Second Swing, though, both the knee joint and the kwa open and close (bend and straighten). This pumps the synovial fluid in the hip joint and releases a very powerful rising current of chi from the earth, feet, and legs that is pumped into the upper body organs, joints and brain.

Guidelines for Learning the Leg Swings

- ### Open and Close the Kwa

  Try to open and close both sides of the kwa with all your weight on only one leg as shown in Figure 13-1 and also with your weight evenly distributed on both legs as shown in Figure 13-2. To close the kwa, sink and squeeze down on the kwa muscles. This decreases the space between the vertebrae of the lower spine *(Figures 13-1A and 13-2A)*. To open the kwa, push or pump up the kwa muscles. This increases the space between the vertebrae *(Figures 13-1B and 13-2B)*.

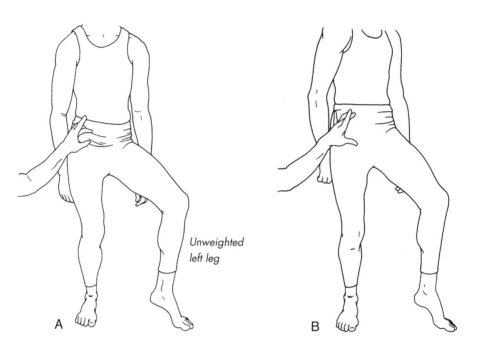

Unweighted left leg

A

B

A) Kwa closed (weight here is 100 percent on right leg). B) Kwa open (weight here is 100 percent on right leg).

Figure 13-1

- ### Only Sink to 70 Percent of Your Physical Capacity

  By practicing in this fashion, your legs and knees will get stronger without risking damage. If you go lower than 70 percent, you may overstrain and injure yourself. Take it slow and easy, and gradually your body will soften up.

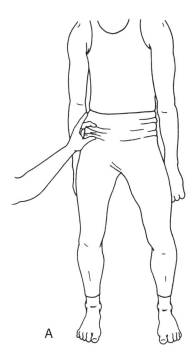 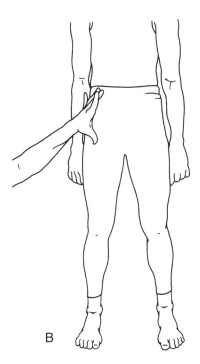

A   B

A) Kwa closed, weight evenly distributed on both legs. B) Kwa open, weight evenly distributed on both legs.
These two actions together are also called bending and stretching the kwa.

Figure 13-2

• Knee Pain Is a Warning Sign

Any pain you might feel in your knees definitely indicates that a correction is in order. First, try standing higher, as you may be re-activating an old injury that you had not paid any attention to, or may not even have realized was there. Make sure when you sink that your knee and ankle are aligned and that you are turning your thighs in conjunction with your waist. Check that your lower back is straight. Make sure that the back of both knees open on opening moves.

• Feel the Chi Spiral Up Inside Your Body

Make sure that the turning in the third swing twists the lower internal organs and that this spiraling energy continues through the center of the body and up to the chest, lungs, neck and directly into the brain. For purposes of this exercise, the brain will be considered part of the upper internal organs.

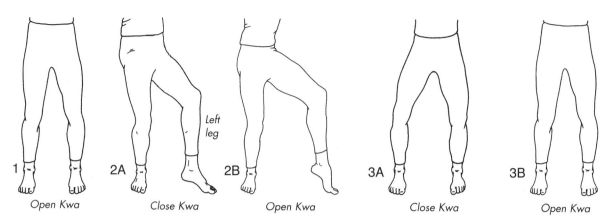

| Open Kwa | Close Kwa | Open Kwa | Close Kwa | Open Kwa |

The Third Swing. This movement is a continuous flow. Positions shown are transitional guides, not static endpoints.
Step 1: Weight equally distributed on both legs; body faces front. Open kwa and shift weight 100 percent to right leg.
Step 2: A) Pivot to left while you simultaneously sink, close kwa, lift left foot and allow left hip and leg to swing. End with ball of foot touching the ground. B) Open kwa.
Step 3. A) Lift your left foot, pivot back to center, close kwa, put foot down, and shift weight to be evenly distributed on both legs. B) Stretch legs and open kwa.

Figure 13-3

1. Begin with Feet Parallel, Kwa Open

Begin with your legs evenly weighted, knees slightly bent, feet parallel and about-shoulder width apart *(Figure 13-3 1)*. Keep your arms down and relaxed. Feel your body weight sinking easily through both legs from hip to ankle to earth. Shift your weight 100 percent to your right leg, as the kwa and the legs slightly open and stretch.

2. Pivot Left: Weight 100 Percent on Right Leg

Lift your left foot and start to pivot to the left, as in the Second Swing, but also sink your body by closing/bending your kwa and right knee *(Figure 13-3 2A)*. As you complete the turn to the left, touch the ground with the ball of your left foot and then open your kwa. Do not straighten your right leg—it remains bent at more or less the same angle *(Figure 13-3 2B)*. Make sure the pumping of the kwa is clear and deliberate.

3. Pivot Back to Center

Lift your left foot and, as you pivot back to center, the kwa closes, the hips sink, and the legs slightly bend as the weight shifts to both feet and is distributed 50/50 *(Figure 13-3 3A)*. Then, open the kwa and knees to straighten and stretch the legs and

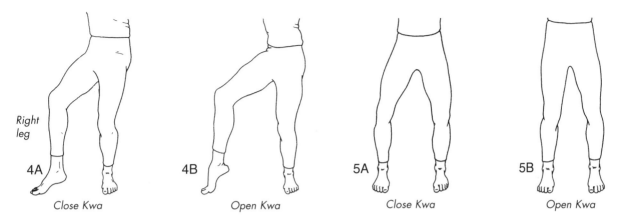

*Right
leg*

4A — Close Kwa

4B — Open Kwa

5A — Close Kwa

5B — Open Kwa

*Step 4: A) Shift weight 100 percent to left leg. Then pivot to right while you simultaneously sink, close kwa, lift right
foot and allow right hip and leg to swing. End with ball of right foot touching the ground. B) Open kwa.*
*Step 5: A) Lift your right foot, pivot back to center, close kwa, put foot down and shift weight to be evenly
distributed on both legs. B) Rise as you stretch legs and open kwa.*

Figure 13-3 (continued)

hips upward *(Figure 13-3 3B)*. Feel the movement of energy moving from the earth to
feet to hips to upper body as you stand up. Most of the vertical movement upward
should be caused by your kwa opening, not your knees.

4. Pivot Right: Weight 100 Percent on Left Leg

As you finish opening, shift your weight 100 percent to the left leg. Now let your body
weight sink easily through both legs from hip to ankle to earth, close your kwa and left
knee and begin to pivot to the right *(Figure 13-3 4A)*. As you complete the pivot to the
right, touch the ground with the ball of your right foot and then open the kwa *(Figure
13-3 4B)*. Do not straighten your left leg—it remains bent at the same angle.

5. Pivot Back to Center

This is a repeat of Step 2 on the opposite side.

6. Repeat Entire Cycle

Repeat entire cycle until it becomes comfortable. *(Figures 13-3 1 to 13-3 5B)*. It will
take time for this movement to become fluid, as most people have let their pelvis "rust"
and stiffen.

Lesson 2 Preparatory Arm Exercises

In the Third Swing, the hands, shoulders and shoulder blades are rotated to their maximum. As with any stretching exercise, it takes time to reach full extension, so here are a few preliminary exercises to start with before attempting the actual swing movement.

1. Two-Partner Exercise to Test if Your Arms Flop Freely

With your arms extended to the front, have a partner hold your arms at the wrist and forearm. Now release any tension in your arms and have your partner bring your arms down to your side. Most people find it very difficult to release control of their arms, so have your partner move your arms an inch or two at a time at first and then gradually increase the distance, until he or she can freely and randomly move your arm anywhere from your head to your knees without any help or resistance on your part. Your entire arm should become a floppy dead weight.

After mastering this exercise, you should be able to raise your hands over your head and drop them below your knees in a totally relaxed fashion. For some people, it may take an hour or two to put this idea into practice. Tension is an easy habit to acquire. Once tension is accumulated and stored in the body it is often difficult to release, but if you are gentle and patient with yourself, it can be done. You will incorporate the arm dropping into Step 3 of these preparatory exercises.

2. Rotate Arm and Shoulder

The footwork for this exercise is the same as for the Second Swing. With the weight on the right foot and waist facing to the left, place the right hand approximately shoulder height in front with the thumb facing the ceiling and the elbow bent. The tip of the elbow should point to the ground, and the arm should be extended and on the centerline of the body. The left arm and hand are held the same as the right—thumb up and shoulder height—and extended to the rear *(Figure 13-4A)*.

With the waist turned as far to the right as is comfortable (keep the head in alignment with the waist—the nose, solar plexus, belly button and groin should be in a straight line), slowly begin to rotate the hands. Maintaining the bend in the elbows, rotate the forearms so that the thumbs first point to the floor, as far as they can comfortably go, and then turn them back to their original position.

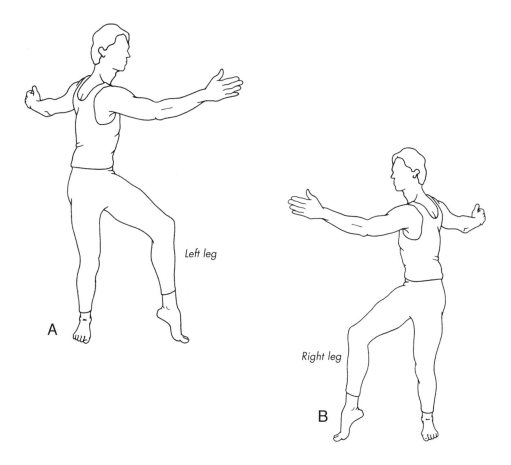

Rotate your thumb up to down and back again in both these stances.
Figure 13-4

Continue this until you have a clear sense of what it feels like for the forearms and, over time, upper arms to rotate, and especially what it feels like to have the thumb point straight up.

Repeat this on the opposite side with the arms and legs reversed *(Figure 13-4B)*.

3. Raise Arms and Let Them Fall Freely

Raise both arms over your head, palms facing forward and then let them fall *(Figure 13-5)*. As they fall, they will naturally rotate so the palms face backward *(Figure 13-6)*. Do not throw the arms down, push them down, or force them down in any way. Just let them go completely, as if the strings of a puppet were cut. Release all control and let them drop naturally.

An indication that this exercise is being done correctly is the sensation of the arms bouncing a little bit when they reach the bottom and naturally swinging back up. It is useful to practice this for ten minutes or more, unless you are very relaxed. If you are very tense, you may need to practice this particular exercise for several hours over many practice sessions before progressing to the next section.

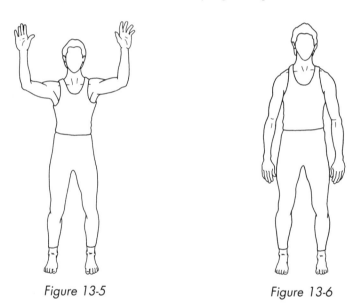

Figure 13-5   Figure 13-6

Lesson 3 The Five-Part Movement
of the Third Swing

1. Facing Center, Raise Arms Above Head

Stand with the feet shoulder-width apart and parallel to each other, body facing forward. Raise both arms over your head, palms facing forward, fingertips toward the sky. The knees and kwa are open *(Figure 13-5)*.

2. Drop Arms, Rotate Hips to Left, Swing Arms Up

Shift weight to the right leg and then pivot to the left, as you learned in Lesson 1. Simultaneously, close your kwa and let the hands drop, as though they had been held by puppet strings that were suddenly cut *(Figure 13-7)*.

With the ball of your left foot having touched the ground and arms facing downward, open your kwa but do not straighten your leg *(Figure 13-8)*. Allow the energy generated by the dropping of the arms and the opening of the kwa to lift the arms.

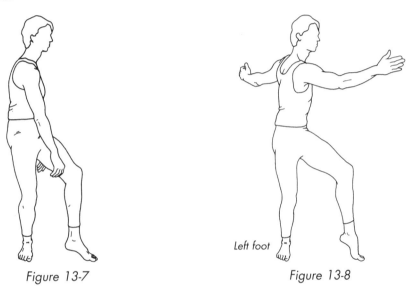

Left foot

Figure 13-7   Figure 13-8

Rotate the hands so that both are thumbs up, with the right hand on the center-line in front and the left hand to the rear. Depending upon how much tension has been released from the arms, the degree of turn in the hips, and especially how much the kwa opens, the hands may finish anywhere from navel height to above the head. The height the arms rise is the height to which energy travels up the body. Do not force your arms upward—that will only stop the flow of chi. Just let them rise as far as they naturally go without independently moving your arms.

Beginners will most likely be quite tense, and the arms will rise correspondingly little. With practice, and the gradual release of tension, the hip will turn more freely, the shoulders rotate further, the kwa open more, and the hands will go higher and higher, until they finally swing up in the air vertically. The legs go through a similar process, bending only slightly at first, but increasing until a deep squat is possible.

An important safety rule: When beginning this exercise, find out how far you can squat and turn, and then only squat and turn about half that amount. Slowly, over many weeks, increase to 70 percent of your capacity, but never exceed that amount. In the West, we do not squat to go to the toilet, so the ligaments of most our knees are not very flexible. Therefore, it is prudent and vitally important that the strength of the knees be increased gradually. Under no circumstances, even if your body is very loose, exceed this 70 percent rule. This exercise includes a torquing action that has few Western equivalents, so be slow, gradual, and gentle so that you do not hurt yourself by being overly zealous.

3. Drop Arms, Rotate Hips and Face Center, Swing Arms Up

- Bring the legs back to parallel, weight 50/50, by closing the kwa and pivoting the hips back to the center. Drop the arms simultaneously *(Figure 13-9)*.

- Open the kwa and straighten legs to propel your arms upward *(Figure 13-10)*.

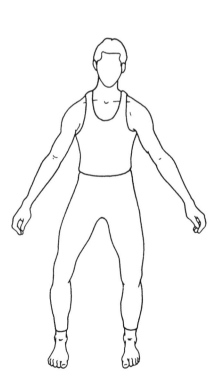

Figure 13-9

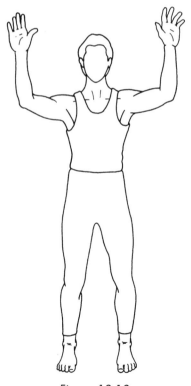

Figure 13-10

Turning back to the center creates centrifugal force, and it is this force, in combination with the opening of the kwa and straightening of the legs, which raises the arms back to their original position. Once again, do not use any voluntary muscular lifting action. In the same way the arms are released to drop, they are released to swing back up. As the body rises, the legs straighten, the kwa continues to lengthen, and the spine and neck raise. The arms rotate back to their original position, so that by the time the body finishes its motion the hands are shoulder-width apart with the palms facing forward and the fingertips lengthening out.

4. Drop Arms, Rotate Hips to Right, Swing Arms Up

Now repeat the same procedure described in step 2 while rotating your hips in the opposite direction (*Figures 13-11* and *13-12*).

5. Drop Arms, Rotate Hips to Center, Swing Arms Up

Repeat Step 3 by turning from the opposite side (*See Figures 13-9* and *13-10*).

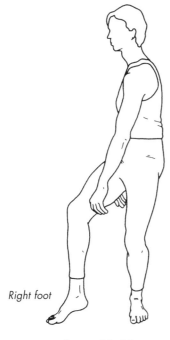

Right foot

Figure 13–11

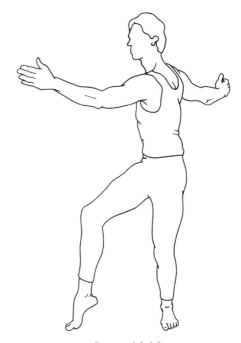

Figure 13-12

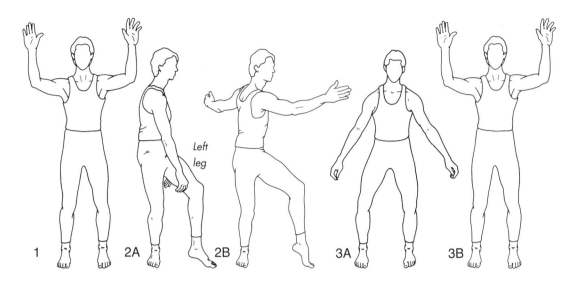

The Third Swing. This movement is a continuous flow. Positions shown are transitional guides, not static end points.

Step 1: Weight equally distributed on both legs; body faces front; arms up as shown.

Step 2: A) Shift weight 100 percent to right leg. Then pivot to left and simultaneously sink, close your kwa, lift your left foot, drop your arms and allow left hip and leg to swing. End with ball of foot touching the ground. B) Open kwa to propel arms up as shown.

Step 3. A) Lift your left foot and pivot back to center, close kwa, drop arms, put left foot down and shift weight to be evenly distributed on both legs. B) Stretch legs and open kwa to propel arms up as shown.

Figure 13-13

6. Practice the Third Swing as a Continuous Movement *(Figures 13-13 1-5B).*

Guidelines for the Third Swing

1. The Rising and Sinking Opens the Macrocosmic Orbit

The opening of the legs and kwa and the lifting of the arms naturally will cause the spine to straighten and energy and blood to rise up the inside of the legs and the back of the torso, neck and head. The lowering and closing of the arms, legs, and waist will cause the energy and blood to move down the front of the forehead, face, neck, and torso and outside of the legs. Together, these actions vigorously circulate the body's energy along what is called the large heavenly, or macrocosmic, orbit.

2. Hands Will Swing Higher with Practice

Over time, tension will progressively release from your arms and you will be able to open your kwa more strongly. As this happens, the faster and more easily your arms

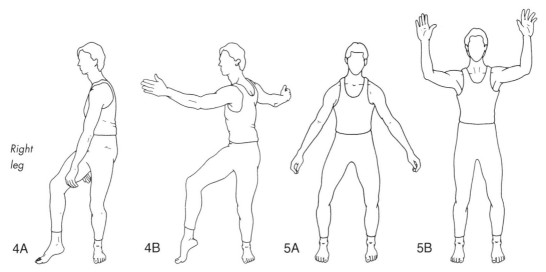

Right leg

4A   4B   5A   5B

Step 4: A) Shift weight 100 percent to left leg. Then pivot to right and simultaneously sink, close your kwa, lift your right foot, drop arms and allow right hip and leg to swing. End with ball of right foot touching the ground. B) Open kwa to propel arms up as shown.

Step 5: A) Lift your right foot and pivot back to center, close kwa, drop arms, put right foot down and shift weight to be evenly distributed on both legs. B) Stretch legs and open kwa to propel arms up as shown.

Figure 13-13 (continued)

will let go and bend and the more strongly your arms will bounce upwards at the end of the downward movement. Eventually, you will feel a strong connection between the opening and closing of your kwa and your arm movements. The closing of the kwa will pull your hands down and the opening of the kwa will push them up.

As the hands reach higher, different organs will benefit. When the hands reach the level of the heart and lungs it is these that will benefit, and as the hands ascend even higher, the energy will flow more and more into the brain.

3. Using Effort to Swing Arms Stifles Chi Flow

If, however, you use your muscular strength to independently raise and lower the arms, the circulation of energy and blood to your spine, heart, lungs and brain will be only minimally increased. You will be doing a purely physical exercise, not one that will amplify your chi.

4. Lift Your Head Gently

It is easy to let the head fall forward during this exercise. This will tighten the neck and shoulders, and impede the swinging of the arms. So remember to keep the head gently lifted off the spine.

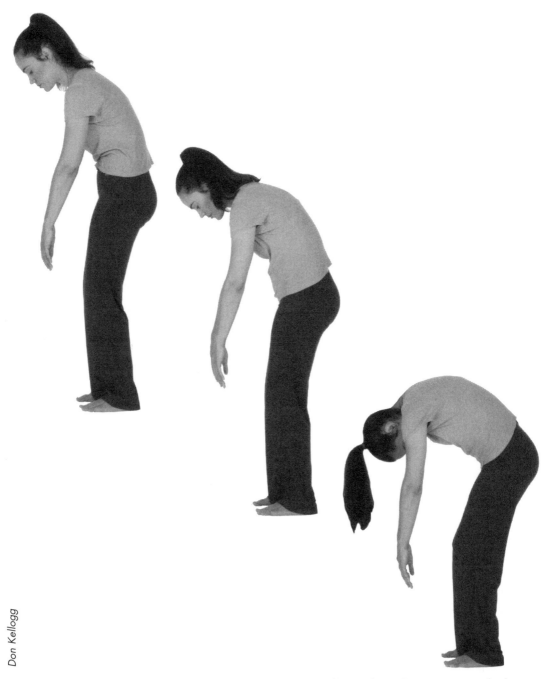

Don Kellogg

The Spine Stretch is an exercise unique to Taoism. Besides making the spine more limber, this exercise begins the process of fully activating the chi of the spine and brain, which is essential for all advanced qigong and other Taoist movement practices.

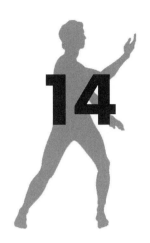

14 The Taoist Spine Stretch

A Supple Spine Is the Backbone of Good Health

In many ways, the Taoist Spine Stretch is probably the single most important technique in this book. In America, back and neck pain necessitates huge amounts of health care services. Such pain may be the result of sedentary work and/or enormous mental tension. Even if you do not attempt the other core qigong exercises presented in previous chapters, you can benefit greatly from doing the Taoist Spine Stretch.

The Spine Stretch has been used to help "incurably" bad backs and can be done by anyone, even those who have severe back problems or are wheelchair bound.

The methodology of the Spine Stretch, which derives from classical Taoist body practices and which is integral to the performance of tai chi chuan and the other internal martial arts, is quite different from the common back stretches found in Western exercise or yoga classes. Common back stretches essentially employ a rolling motion, where from a standing position, the head and neck, then the chest, then the mid and lower back, collapse as the upper body moves progressively closer and closer to the floor. This is the exact opposite of what you will be doing in the Taoist Spine Stretch.

First you will learn to feel your spine and distinguish the muscles from the actual vertebrae. Most people can barely feel their back except when it aches. In fact, many people in the West cannot even feel the muscles of their back.

Next you will learn to slowly bend from the kwa while keeping your spine and head straight.

Finally you will learn to release tension from within the vertebrae, while you are both bending and straightening. This exercise will help strengthen your legs and hips, without putting any pressure on your back.

Your alignments do not have to be perfect to do this exercise. People with severe back problems should use very small movements, perhaps learning to do this stretch while sitting, paying close attention to the recommended warm-ups, and not bending the spine at all at first.

More advanced techniques for doing the Spine Stretch (for those with more experience in the core exercises in this book, or other Taoist energy practices) are found later in this chapter.

Remember that in all qigong, first you learn physical movements, then you add components that involve the flow of energy. In the view of the Taoist masters, "If properly nurtured, small acorns over time grow into great oaks."

The Posterior and Anterior Sides of the Spine

The *posterior* side of the vertebrae faces behind you and is what most identify as their backbone. Energetically it governs the ability of the spine to bend as well as the ability of the legs to bend and to sit down. For most, the back of the spine is relatively easy to feel because we constantly press it against the back of chairs and lie on it all the time. The *anterior* or front side of the vertebrae energetically governs the ability of the spine to stand up from a lying or seated position and to lift upwards and bear weight. The anterior side of the spine is relatively more difficult for most to feel and locate by awareness alone, as it faces our belly and navel and is hidden inside the body. For many the front of the spine is challenge to feel; both because normally nothing obviously presses on it and it is rarely mentioned as something we should be able to feel.

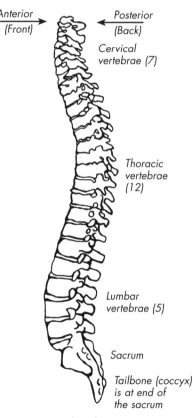

Anterior (Front)   Posterior (Back)

Cervical vertebrae (7)

Thoracic vertebrae (12)

Lumbar vertebrae (5)

Sacrum

Tailbone (coccyx) is at end of the sacrum

Spinal Column

Figure 14-1

The posterior and anterior side of each vertebra can open and close. Think of two children's building blocks, one on top of the other. You can open and close the space between these blocks from either the front or back end. The same is true of your vertebrae. Moreover, each vertebra can open and close independently of any other vertebrae, without relying on any external movement. Gaining control of the movements of the spine and the energy they generate is an integral part of neigong (see Chapter 15). From the viewpoint of qigong, the spine is primarily an energetic transfer conduit, rather than just a series of bones and other physical structure such as fluids, nerves, muscle, membranes and connective tissues. From this perspective, how you induce energy to flow in the spine using the posterior and anterior side of the spine is as important as the fact that you are physically stretching it.[1]

Spine Warm-ups

Warm-up 1: Feel Your Spine

Lie on the ground with your knees up in the air, so that the whole length of your back is more or less touching the ground. Begin to take very deep breaths, until it feels as though your breath is extending back to the spine and the muscles surrounding it, including the kidneys (see p. 84). Take a few minutes, until you can use your breath to feel all the vertebrae along the back of your spine (its posterior side).

What you are attempting to do now is to get a sense of the difference between your back muscles and the vertebrae of your spine. By pressing up with your legs and lifting your bottom, or lifting up your head and neck and shoulders, you want to make each small section of your spine touch the floor in an isolated fashion, so that you can clearly differentiate the sections of the spine. If you have a back problem do this on mats or thick carpet to protect your spine.

Warm-up 2: Bend Only at the Kwa

This exercise can be done standing or while sitting in a chair. Over time, you will want to do this exercise standing.

Review the principles and alignments of how to stand (pp. 96–104). Your alignments do not have to be perfect. Do your best to stand with your feet parallel, shoulder-width apart,

---

[1] The Spine Stretch is a preliminarily exercise for more advanced neigong techniques taught in the author's Bend the Bow Spinal Qigong program (see Appendix G).

hands at your sides, without any of your joints locked. Keep your buttocks tucked under, so that your lower back is straight.

The two purposes of this warm-up are to make your legs and hips strong enough to support the weight of your back and neck, and to help your feet to gain the ability to root into the ground. In order to stabilize your balance, you will usually need to practice this warm-up 10 to 20 times over a few days, or much time and energy will be wasted trying to maintain balance during the more complicated Spine Stretch itself. A half an hour to an hour of this preliminary warm-up can save many hours of confusion, as well as prevent strain on the lower back.

1. From a standing position, bend forward from the kwa, while keeping your spine absolutely straight. Some may be able to bend forward only an inch or so; others might bend until they feel their spine parallel with the floor. Only bend forward as far as is comfortable, staying within 70 percent of your capacity. There should be no strain on the back when you do this since you are only bending at the kwa.
   - If you are standing, try not to let your tailbone move backward.
   - The movement of the torso must originate from the kwa and not from your back muscles, head or neck.
   - The spine does not bend or twist in any way. Treat it as though it were a stable rod from the top of the neck to the tailbone. Be sure not to tense the back muscles while doing this.
   - While standing, the feet do not move and the shins and thighs remain parallel to each other, with the perineum open. Keeping the feet still reduces the chance of the knees bowing in or out.
   - Any wobble or feeling of being off balance means that you are bending too far forward.

2. Rise up from the kwa, keeping the back straight with the tailbone unmoving throughout. Once you are comfortable doing the kwa bend, try to feel the weight of your torso clearly descending through your legs into your feet while bending. When rising, try and feel the strength rising from your feet, through your legs to your kwa. Take as much pressure off your back as possible and put it on the kwa and your legs.

   If you can, work with a partner, who can make sure that you are not arching or bending your back or neck in any way. It is easy to think you are not arching your back when in fact you are. Feedback from a partner can be useful in this situation.

Lesson 1 The Taoist Spine Stretch— First Half

The critical component of the first half of the Taoist Spine Stretch is the ability to put your mind inside your body and release any strength, tension, or chi blockage, as you let go of muscular volition and control of your back muscles. In other words, it is necessary to target your mind on a part of your body and then let go of as much accumulated control or holding as best as you can, (that is, dissolve the energy in each inter-vertebral space—"ice to water to gas."

A good way to get a feeling for what this is like is to hold your hand in a fist without squeezing or tightening it. Then mentally release everything that allows it to be in a fist until it opens, and then release all sense of physicality into the air away from your body. This can also be practiced by closing your eyes and relaxing them open, curling your toes and relaxing them open, etc. Become aware of the internal processes that allow this kind of relaxation to take place. At first, only use this technique on places that easily open and close and, at least initially, avoid places of chronic tension in your body. Build success in easier places in your body before getting to the work you most need to do.

1. Mentally Release Tension in the Vertebrae at the Base of the Spine, from the Posterior (Back) Side of the Vertebrae

Stand with the feet between hip- and shoulder-width apart, whichever is the most comfortable. Keep your arms and hands relaxed *(Figure 14-4A)*.

Next, bend forward at the kwa only as far as is comfortable.

2. First Learn to Work with Groups of Vertebrae, Then Individual Ones

When you work by yourself in the beginning, it is quite natural to be able to feel only groups of vertebrae rather than each one separately. For example, some people will feel two to four, or four to six vertebrae at a time. When following these instructions, first just release and open whatever group of vertebrae you can feel—be it one, two, four, or even eight vertebrae.

Over time, the size of the group may decrease, and within a year of practice, you should be able to feel individual vertebrae.

A) In the posture shown in Figure 14-4A, begin by mentally releasing all the

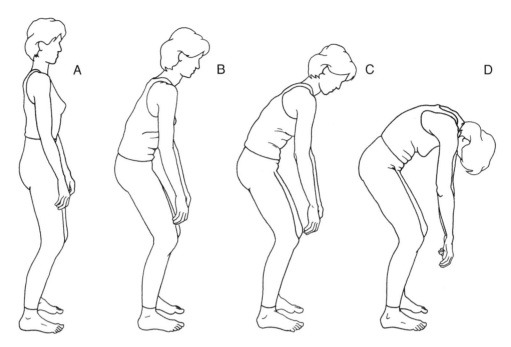

The Spine Stretch—First Half. A) Starting posture: Feet parallel, back straight, head lifted, chest dropped, belly relaxed, shoulders rounded. B), C) & D) Gradually release vertebrae from bottom to top, bending forward as each release is achieved. Release from the posterior (back) side of vertebrae.

Figure 14-4

tension between the first five vertebrae above your sacrum up to your fifth lumbar on the posterior side of the spine (see *Figure 14-1*). Do not release the tension found above the fifth vertebra—let it remain there for the moment.

The fifth lumbar is the main weight-bearing vertebra of the spine. It is where the curve in the lower back is most pronounced. It also is the place where people are most likely to experience low back pain.

B) While bending at the kwa, let gravity gently and naturally pull this first group of vertebrae slightly apart. This will release any remaining tension by increasing the space between each disc of as many vertebrae you are choosing to release (*Figure 14-4B*). Your body may be so bound up that it takes a few weeks before you can get an actual physical separation of the vertebrae, but you must continue to work on this area with your mind until some sort of release is felt in the nerves or chi.

Over time, the release of the nerves will cause the muscles to let go and allow the vertebrae to separate slightly. In order for the body to bend at all, the vertebrae must release and separate on some level, although it can be so slight as to be unnoticeable—what you want to achieve is to gradually increase this stretch.

As you do the Spine Stretch over the next few weeks or months, gravity will help increase the distance between this first group of vertebrae and the next group; or, as you become more experienced, between each individual vertebra. The degree of release will increase with time.

3. Release and Stretch the Next Group of Vertebrae

Next, move your mind to next group of vertebrae on the posterior side of the spine that are just above the ones you have just worked on and released *(Figure 14-4C and D)*. First mentally release any tension. Then again, let gravity gently open these vertebrae. Again, above these vertebrae, nothing moves, bends, or twists in any fashion. Your spine only bends slightly at the place where you have already released your vertebrae. Then proceed upwards on your spine, group by group. Over time, you will find that the group of vertebrae you can feel may go from six to four; or four to two, or that you can sometimes feel a release in only one vertebra before going on to a new group. Eventually you will be able to release one vertebra at a time.

It is very helpful to have a partner place his or her finger(s) on the group of vertebrae you are trying to release to help direct your attention to the location.

Continue this process, releasing one vertebra or group of vertebrae at a time. Every time you release a vertebra you may further release any of the vertebrae below it, but you must keep bound and unmoving the vertebrae above the one you are working on. As you approach the neck, it will be very difficult to keep your head from flopping. Be aware of this tendency, and have a partner help you correct this by holding his or her arm in front of your nose. Your partner will immediately let you know when you have bent your upper spine and neck prematurely.

4. Progressively Release the Shoulder and Arm Joints as You Release the Cervical Vertebrae

Releasing from the big vertebra at the bottom of the neck (the seventh cervical) through to the atlas at the base of the head (the first cervical) proves to be the most difficult for the majority of people. When releasing from the seventh to the first cervical vertebrae, progressively allow the joints of the shoulders, elbows, wrists, palms, and fingers to open up and release one by one. By the time the atlas has released, the finger joints should also be completely released. This will improve the nerve and chi flow between the spine, arms and fingertips.

5. Release the Skull Plates

After releasing the atlas, to the best of your ability begin to release the skull plates. The human skull is not one bone, but rather a number of plates joined together by sutures. These plates are capable of being released through voluntary action. When the spine, neck, and skull plates release, the nerve and chi flow in the body, as well as the strength of the cerebrospinal pump, will be greatly improved.

Lesson 2 The Taoist Spine Stretch— Second Half

The spine has two main functions. One is to bend and flex (which has been covered in the first part of this exercise). The second function of the spine is to lift, so that we may stand erect. It is this second function that is addressed in the second half of the spinal stretch.

1. Open, Lift and Lengthen the Anterior (Front) Side of the Spine as You Unbend and Straighten Upwards

At this point, your legs are still shoulder-width apart and your spine, head, and arms are totally released. Again, work from the bottom toward the top, leaving the vertebrae above the area of focus unchanged. This same process should be repeated for each vertebra (or group of vertebrae) until you reach your neck *(Figure 14-5A-D)*.

In the first half of the stretch, the back (posterior side) of the spine is especially lengthened and separated from the vertebrae below it. In the second half, as you are coming up, it is the inner or anterior side of the spine that is especially lengthened, lifted and focused upon.

2. Unbend and Raise the Spine, One Vertebra at a Time

Proceed to the next two higher vertebrae with your mind. Then physically lengthen and lift them straight up, leaving everything above the third vertebra to the top of your head still totally released and floppy. Again, it is very useful to have a

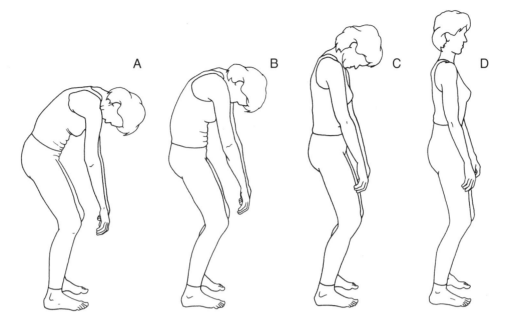

The Spine Stretch—Second Half. A) Posture upon completion of first half (you are bent all the way forward). B), C) & D) As you stand erect, open the anterior (front) side of the spine from bottom to top. Opening means lifting each vertebra in the front (vertebrae are already opened in the back from the first part of the stretch).

Figure 14-5

partner put a finger between the two vertebrae you are working on, so that the area concerned can be felt more easily and more awareness can be brought to it. Your partner should keep a hand on the back of your neck to help stop your upper back and neck from moving backward or straightening before their time as these vertebrae must remain completely floppy and released. In the same way, during the first half of the exercise, your partner, to help boost your awareness, kept a hand in front of your nose to keep your neck and upper back from relaxing and dropping forward before their time.

3. Avoid Stiffening the Neck

It will be when you reach the middle of the upper back that problems will almost certainly arise, and the neck will have the greatest tendency to stiffen and raise or bend backwards. This is the equivalent to where, in the first half of the Spine Stretch, when bending the spine forward, your neck and upper back may have wanted to prematurely release downward.

4. Take Extra Care Raising the Neck and Stretching the Skull

The most important areas to consider are the opening and straightening of the vertebrae from the base of the neck to the base of the skull, and the opening of the plates of the skull. Paying extra attention to these areas prevents energy from getting stuck in the spine. From the seventh cervical vertebra to the plates of your skull, in progressive increments, you will simultaneously raise your neck and head higher and gently push open your arm joints to your fingertips, one by one, just as you released them at the end of the downward bend.

Guidelines for Practicing the Taoist Spine Stretch

1. Practice with a Partner First

Your partner's hands on your back will help you begin to become aware of and feel each vertebra of the spine as a separate entity.

2. Learn to Separate Groups of Vertebrae, Then Individual Ones

When you work by yourself in the beginning, it is quite natural to only be able to feel large parts of your back as a unit. For most people, the unit of sensation is anywhere from four to six vertebrae, though within a year most people are able to feel their vertebrae one by one. So at first, just release and open whatever your unit of sensation is—be it one, two, four, or even eight vertebrae.

3. Maximum of Three Spine Stretches per Practice Session

Under no circumstance do more than three Spine Stretches in any one practice session. This is a safety precaution against overstraining. Also, after three Spine Stretches, the effectiveness as regards the time spent and benefits of doing more Spine Stretches radically diminishes. If you feel as though your spine really wants a good workout, simply spend more time on each Spine Stretch rather than increasing the number of repetitions. You could also practice more than one session a day as long as there is at least a four-hour interval between sessions.

4. Avoid Sudden Increases in Practice Times

If you practice these exercises every day or every other day, which is the most beneficial way to do them, and for some reason your life situation prevents practice for a week or so, do not try to make up for lost time. Do a little bit less than you were practicing before your layoff. Increase incrementally with each practice session. In this way, you will avoid jarring your nervous system or overstraining your muscles.

5. Focus on Releasing the Vertebrae, Not on Stretching

It is important to realize that it is not a requirement of the Taoist Spine Stretch to bend very low. This is not a high school gym exercise. You want your spine to regain the soft, natural flexibility of that of a child, but this process takes time and cannot be rushed. It is not the stretch that is important at first, but your ability to place your mind into the vertebrae that you want to release. Make sure you do not overstrain or fight through pain or an injury—go slow and be patient. Over time, you will gain increasing control over your spine and help it to become more flexible.

Doing the Taoist Spine Stretch While Sitting

Although many qigong practices are primarily done moving, they can also be done sitting, standing, lying down and during human interactions, such as conversation or sex. The Taoist Spine Stretch can be also done while sitting, and is useful for anyone who engages in prolonged sitting, for example, at work, school or during meditation.

The basic method for doing a sitting Spine Stretch is very similar to that of the standing Spine Stretch. Make sure you understand the process by reviewing the instructions earlier in this chapter. Pay particular attention to how and why the posterior and anterior parts of individual or groups of the spinal vertebrae separate, move and stretch as you bend forward in the first half of the stretch and straighten in the second half.

Sitting Spine Stretch Warm-ups

Review Spine Warm-up 2 in this chapter and the principles and alignments of how to sit (pp.104–107). While sitting, do a few kwa bends as a warm-up. Keep your torso and head upright; let your body incline forward and then return to its original position.

Remember: a kwa bend originates the movement of the torso from the kwa and not your back muscles, head or neck. Keep your lower back straight while solely using the impetus of your legs and kwa to both lean forward and straighten your back. Keep your feet firmly planted, solidly contacting the floor when bending or straightening. See if you can feel the weight of your torso clearly descending through your legs into your feet while bending; when rising, try and feel the strength rising from your feet, through your legs to your kwa. Take as much pressure off your back as possible and put it on the kwa and your legs.

Adhere to the 70 percent rule to avoid back strain. Try to make sure that the strength to raise and lower your back derives from pushing up from your feet, through your legs and kwa to your spine, and not from your back muscles.

If you have physical difficulties and must sit, or are in a wheelchair, and cannot physically use your legs to push up from the ground, engage your kwa rather than depending in any way on your back muscles. This will help avoid any back strain at all.

The Sitting Spine Stretch

1. Bend your spine slightly forward. Go to the base of your spine at the tailbone and first mentally release tension in the bottom vertebrae as best as you can. Then focus on letting gravity release and open the posterior sides of your vertebrae one by one or in small groups. Begin at your tailbone and progress to the top of your neck *(Figure 14-6)*.

2. While still bent forward, as you begin to straighten your spine, focus your attention on the bottom of the anterior side of your vertebrae at your tailbone and sacrum. Release and open successive anterior sides of your vertebrae either individually or in small groups *(Figure 14-7)*.

3. If one side of your body is more contracted than the other, place more emphasis on pushing up from the kwa that is on the contracted side.

The Next Level of the Spine Stretch

Once you are comfortable with the physical movements of the Spine Stretch, either standing or sitting, it is time to begin engaging with some of the dynamics of moving energy from the spine downwards. For this, you need to be able to implement the fundamental

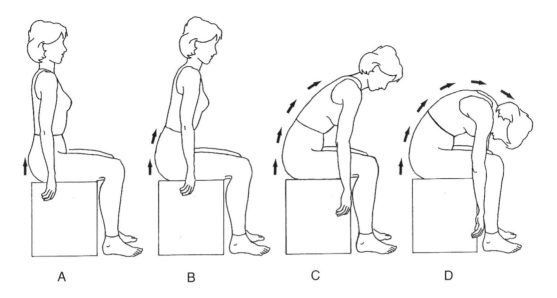

The Sitting Spine Stretch—First Half. A) Starting posture: Feet parallel, back straight, head lifted, chest dropped, belly relaxed, shoulders rounded. B), C) & D) Gradually release vertebrae from bottom to top, bending forward as each release is achieved. Release from the posterior (back) side of vertebrae.

Figure 14-6

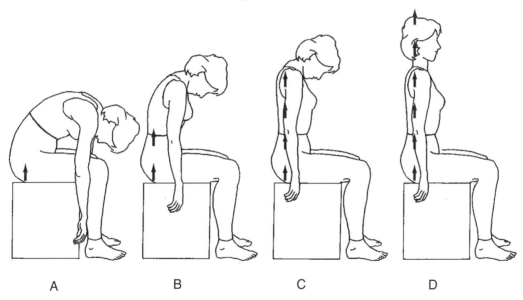

The Sitting Spine Stretch—Second Half. A) Posture upon completion of first half (you are bent all the way forward). B), C) & D) As you stand erect, open the anterior (front) side of the spine from bottom to top. (Opening means lifting each vertebra from the front of the vertebrae. The posterior side of the vertebrae have already been opened from the first part of the stretch).

Figure 14-7

standing techniques, which include sinking your energy, scanning your energy body and the chi dissolving process (see Chapter 7).

Although sinking the chi and dissolving may be used independently, ideally they should be combined to enhance the benefits of the kwa bend or the Spine Stretch. The best strategy for smoothly integrating the two methods is to first sink your chi for a minimum of a month or as long as it takes until by your own standards you feel minimally competent, and only then add dissolving.

As you do the Spine Stretch, you will progressively incorporate these techniques into it. The process of sinking and dissolving does not just apply to the Taoist Spine Stretch. Sinking and dissolving ideally should be used whenever you:

- Feel an alignment that does not go into place easily.
- Experience any persistent pain in your body.
- Encounter an energy blockage or pain when you are doing a qigong or other Taoist energy arts movement.
- Want to encourage more chi to flow in your body.

What is important during this next phase is how much you can relax your nerves and how much chi you can release in the spine.

Advanced Warm-up 1: Feel Your Spine More Precisely

It is important to learn to develop more sensitivity to precisely feeling the vertebrae in the posterior and anterior parts of your spine.

In the Spine Warm-up 1 (p. 217), you learned to differentiate your back muscles from your spine. Now go back and repeat Spine Warm-up 1 and focus your attention on exactly what the posterior and anterior side of each vertebra individually feels like.

Then extend this inner exploration to bringing your awareness to the quality of what the entire vertebra feels like—back, side and front. For this task dissolving the entire vertebra may prove a very powerful and helpful tool.

Next allow your awareness to go further and explore how the anterior side of any vertebrae you choose to feel, in some indefinable way, has a different feeling from the posterior side of the same vertebrae. Something will be different for you—maybe a mood change or feeling of pressure. Be patient, keep searching and do your best to refine this subtle feeling.

Staying relaxed, then experiment with feeling and moving anything inside the abdomen you can (muscles, organs, etc.) until you can detect any part of the anterior side of any spinal vertebrae moving, even if just a little—especially those vertebrae moving up and down vertically, as they come closer together and move apart. Then extend this movement to as many vertebrae as you can. You should not attempt to move your vertebrae sideways.

Advanced Warm-up 2: Kwa Bend—The Next Level

1. Bend from the Kwa

Slowly bend forward from the kwa. As you do so, sink and/or dissolve your chi through your legs. Remember to keep your back straight.

2. Push Up from the Legs

When lifting upwards, gently push up from your feet through the inside of your legs. This will enable you to use the natural strength of your legs to help push up and lift the kwa and the weight of your torso, without putting any weight on your knees. Do this without straightening your legs much and with minimal leg extension. Increased experience with sinking chi and dissolving through the legs makes this progressively effective and easier to do.

3. Sink Your Energy

Next, as you slowly bend down from the kwa, sink and/or dissolve the energy from your entire spine down your legs into the floor. Feel each individual or small group of vertebrae and release any bound energy from them through your legs to the floor. Because the energy of the spine and legs are so interconnected, sometimes also slowing down and dissolving the chi at the place it seems to get stuck in your legs on its downward journey can further release bound energy in the spine either during the kwa bend or in the Spine Stretch itself.

How to Apply Sinking and Dissolving During the Spine Stretch

1. Settling In

Before bending from the kwa, take a few moments to simultaneously sink the chi of your entire spine through your legs to your feet.

2. Sink Your Chi and Release Each Vertebra, One at a Time

A) Bend forward at the kwa. For each individual vertebra sink the chi from that vertebra until the chi reaches your feet and your legs become internally wet (see p. 118). Then continue to sink your chi through your legs during all bending and straightening phases of the Spine Stretch. This will help you to connect your legs to your spine, ground the spine's energy and improve the release of blocked energy within your vertebrae. As best you can, maintain

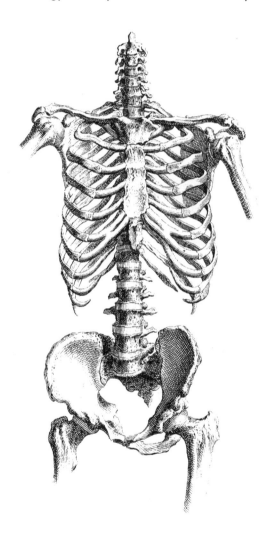

Front of the spine shown in relation to the ribs and the pelvic area

Figure 14-8

a continuous downward wave of sinking chi throughout the entire Spine Stretch, regardless of whether or not you add dissolving to it. Do this until you can release and sink your chi through whichever single vertebra or group of vertebrae you are focusing on during all downward phases of the Spine Stretch. Each time you do the stretch, try to increase the release of bound energy.

B) As you straighten, continue to sink your chi as best as you can. Continue for as long as it takes for your body to acclimatize to sinking before going to the next step. This may take days, weeks, or longer.

3. Both Sink and Dissolve Your Chi

Next, apply releasing, sinking the chi and dissolving techniques together as best you can. When going downwards, first dissolve the vertebrae you are working on to the boundary of your etheric body.

Then sink the dissolved chi of the vertebrae you are working on down to your feet as you bend your kwa slightly and stretch the posterior side of the vertebrae. You can also dissolve this dropping spinal chi wherever it also becomes blocked in your legs, before continuing on and completely sinking the chi to your feet.

When straightening your spine, again dissolve the same vertebrae and sink its chi to your feet, before physically pushing up from your feet, through the inside of your legs to lift your kwa and thereby aid in lifting the vertebrae. Your legs should always remain slightly bent while straightening the spine.

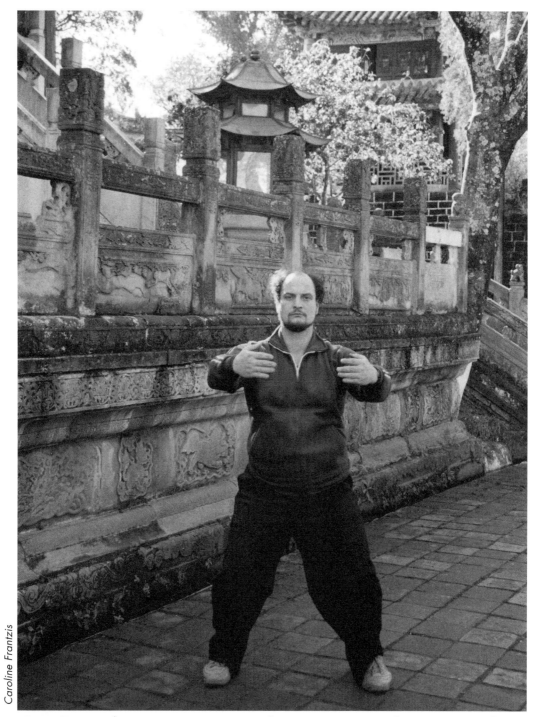

Caroline Frantzis

Bruce Frantzis demonstrates a qigong standing posture at a temple in Kunming, China.

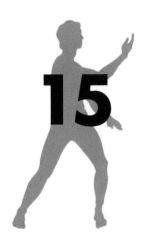

15 Neigong: The Heart of Taoist Energy Practices

Going to the Next Level of Qigong

This chapter will show practitioners of any form of qigong or tai chi where their learning might progress.

Until the past few decades, qigong was only known and understood in China. Today, in the West, the knowledge of the potential of the complete system of qigong is still incomplete.

To many in the West, qigong is merely an Oriental way of doing physical movements; a kind of dance or beautiful movement therapy; or it is a mysterious form of powerful martial art. In China for millennia, the full potential of qigong for the mind, body and spirit has been realized through the practices of neigong.

Intellectual and Embodied Knowledge

There are two kinds of knowledge about body/mind subjects. The first entails only that you intellectually understand the framework within which it exists. The second type of knowledge regarding neigong requires that you experience it in your body. The first kind of knowledge does not require a teacher. The second needs a teacher along with support materials such as this book. In this regard, this chapter serves three audiences:

- The first are intellectually curious readers who have never personally done qigong but would like to know what it is all about. Enough detail is presented on this vast subject so that a coherent picture of its depth and complexity emerges, much of which has previously been unavailable in print. Qigong is shown to be more than merely physical movements, but rather an important way to access your inner ecology through a sophisticated energy technology called neigong.

- The second group consists of practitioners who have learned a little qigong and would like to go further.
- The third audience consists of long-term, more advanced qigong practitioners and teachers. Those who have had the good fortune to have obtained enough authentic experience from qualified teachers can reasonably attempt to do some of the methods mentioned here without needing careful monitoring or the kind of step-by-step instructions contained in other parts of this book. They may also be inspired to seek out fuller knowledge of neigong, so that they can authentically embody it and transfer it to others.

The Next Level of Opening the Energy Gates of Your Body

The next level of the Energy Gates program involves learning more sophisticated aspects of neigong. There are three paths:

- You can be taught specific aspects of neigong to incorporate into the movements you have already learned—standing, Cloud Hands, three swings and the Spine Stretch.
- You can learn more sophisticated standing postures and deeper aspects of movements already learned, such as the Spiraling Energy Body Qigong program (p. 236 and p. 285), which focuses on various components of neigong.
- You can learn entirely new qigong movements, which may make it easier to learn particular components of neigong. Once learned, any aspect of neigong can be used in any Taoist system and has the potential to be adapted for use within other traditions.

Standing Postures

The original Taoist energetic system is composed of approximately 200 static standing postures. It was already well known during the Tang Dynasty, China's Golden Age (A.D. 618–907). All the basic internal energy flows and basic postures of the internal martial arts of tai chi, hsing-i, ba gua and the eight postures of I Chuan are derived from this system. One school of thought in China states that the entire system of qigong can be learned purely through the 200 or so static standing postures. However, the majority opinion is that although standing is immensely valuable, moving and sitting practices are essential to the mix.

What Is a Posture?

The Chinese term *shr*, or "posture" in English, as used in qigong and tai chi is confusing because it fuses two ideas that are normally separated. From a standing qigong perspective, the final pose or position, such as the standing posture shown *(Figure 15-1)* is static. Here the term shr means posture as is understood in English.

In moving qigong, the entire dynamic, continuous motion is also called a posture. However these movements are identified and named only by their final static positions. The different postures within the qigong movements that lead to the final position are not named. For example, both Cloud Hands and each of the three swings are composed of several linked static postures from the original 200 or so postures.

Qualities of the Standing Postures

Going to the next level of standing qigong requires engagement with at least some of the 200 postures.

Standing with your feet parallel and arms at your sides is the easiest and the most energetically neutral of the entire system *(Figure 15-1)*. It is the ideal posture through which to first learn the science of Taoist standing qigong.

The next posture you are likely to learn is standing with your arms at about chest height and rounded, as if you were hugging a tree (see p. 232).

Each of the postures benefits your chi as a whole and is helpful for whatever Taoist practice you choose. However, each posture also has its own distinct function that activates and makes you aware of specific primary chi circuits. Each causes your body to change in specific ways. Each can be used to focus your energy to heal specific issues, develop specific kinds of physical power and release innate abilities.

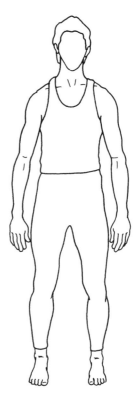

Basic Standing Posture
Figure 15-1

Stances and Arm Positions of the Postures

The 200 or so internal postures are done using three stances:

- The basic stance taught in this book.
- Alternating between your weight being evenly distributed on both legs and turning your hips so all your weight rests on one leg at a time.
- Standing with different proportions of your weight on each leg, often with your feet in nonparallel positions.

The arm and hand positions of the postures have a great degree of variability. Your arms may mirror each other, or each may do something different. Variations include:

- Height of your hands.
- Orientation of your hands vis-à-vis your centerline—hands facing the front, side or back.
- Orientation of your palms and fingers.
- Distance of your hands from your body.

Qigong healers and teachers can teach customized standing postures to correct specific energy imbalances or to bring out potential energies and talents.

Spiraling Energy Body Qigong

Spiraling Energy Body Qigong is Part 2 of Opening the Energy Gates of Your Body Qigong. It is one of the advanced stages of the Frantzis Energy Arts qigong system (see Appendix G). Here, standing qigong, Cloud Hands, the three swings and the Spine Stretch are used for progressively incorporating more components of the neigong system. This course includes additional fundamental theory and specific internal techniques. Other aspects of neigong are initially more easily learned using physical movements different from those in Energy Gates Qigong, such as Gods Playing in the Clouds Qigong.

The 16 Components of the Neigong System

The Taoist science of how energy flows in humans is derived from the 16 components of neigong. Figures 15-2 and 15-3 show the body's energy anatomy.

These are the 16 components:

1. Breathing methods from the simple to the complex.
2. Moving chi along the various ascending, descending and lateral connecting channels within the body.
3. Adjusting body alignments that prevent the flow of chi.
4. Dissolving, releasing and resolving all blockages.
5. Moving chi through all the acupuncture channels, energy gates and points.
6. Bending and stretching soft tissues from the inside out and from the outside in, along the yin and yang acupuncture channels.
7. Openings and closings (pulsing).
8. Working with the energies of your aura or etheric body.
9. Generating circles and spirals of energy inside your body.
10. Absorbing and projecting chi and moving it to any part of your body at will.
11. Awakening and controlling all the energies of your spine.
12. Awakening and using your left and right energy channels.
13. Awakening and using your central energy channel.
14. Developing and using your lower tantien.
15. Developing and using your middle and upper tantien.
16. Integrating and connecting each of the previous 15 components into one unified process.

The order of the 16 neigong components is not fixed or linear, only descriptive. Each component forms a segment of a circle. Just as there is no beginning or end point of a continuously rotating circle, neigong has neither a beginning nor end. Each component catalyzes and influences the others. Every time you revisit any of the components, it becomes possible to attain a deeper, more fulfilling and beneficial level within the component itself and those that precede and follow it. Learning and incorporating aspects of neigong into your practice is what makes qigong an ever-evolving art—one that can engage, interest and inspire you throughout your life.

The Energy Anatomy of the Body
reprinted from *The Power of Internal Martial Arts and Chi*

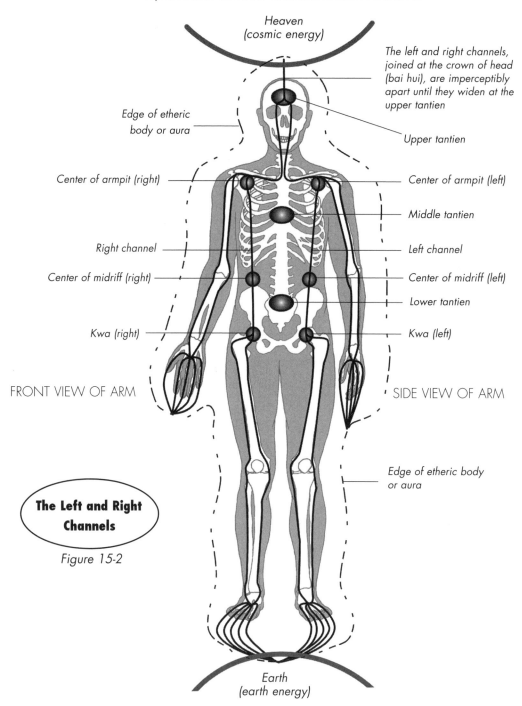

Heaven
(cosmic energy)

The left and right channels,
joined at the crown of head
(bai hui), are imperceptibly
apart until they widen at the
upper tantien

Edge of etheric
body or aura

Upper tantien

Center of armpit (right)

Center of armpit (left)

Middle tantien

Right channel

Left channel

Center of midriff (right)

Center of midriff (left)

Lower tantien

Kwa (right)

Kwa (left)

FRONT VIEW OF ARM

SIDE VIEW OF ARM

Edge of etheric body
or aura

**The Left and Right
Channels**

Figure 15-2

Earth
(earth energy)

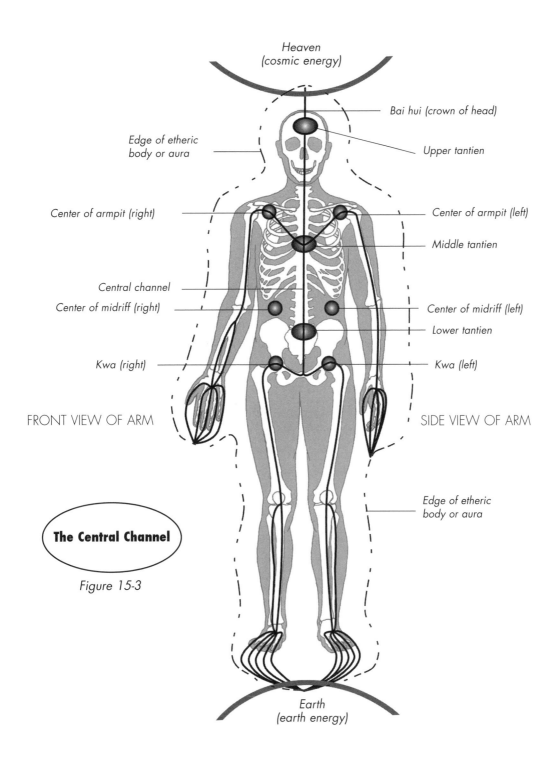

Heaven
(cosmic energy)

Bai hui (crown of head)

Upper tantien

Edge of etheric
body or aura

Center of armpit (right)

Center of armpit (left)

Middle tantien

Central channel

Center of midriff (right)

Center of midriff (left)

Lower tantien

Kwa (right)

Kwa (left)

FRONT VIEW OF ARM

SIDE VIEW OF ARM

Edge of etheric
body or aura

The Central Channel

Figure 15-3

Earth
(earth energy)

The Neigong Continuum of Knowledge

Knowledge has various levels. Both between and within the hundred plus different qigong schools in China, those masters with the higher or highest standards are commonly called "real" while those with lower ones are often called either "ordinary" or unqualified. The ultimate basis of the standard applied is usually how completely each of the 16 neigong components are taught.

Depending on your background and degree of intrinsic interest, what is presented as "real neigong" by any individual or found in any qigong book may be too high a level for some and too low for others.

Learning Real Neigong

Neigong is best learned with a live instructor. The subtleties of its physical and energetic movements are not easily or fully observable in books or videotapes. Energy work can engender both positive and negative states and create strong emotional releases: a good teacher will know how to help you learn to handle them appropriately.

Cheng Man Ching, a famous tai chi instructor who used to live in New York City, put it this way, "Three things are required to attain a high level of embodied success in tai chi or qigong: 1) Having a good teacher; 2) Perseverance and practice; 3) Natural talent. Of the three the most important is a good teacher." Without a good teacher, you can't know how to best apply your perseverance and natural talent and so may, even with the best of intentions, go down the wrong road. Most good teachers have a certain level of natural talent and their insights are valuable to help you bring out yours.

Neigong is more easily written and talked about than learned.

Although the complete neigong system can be made accessible, most people will need copious amounts of practice and repetition to embody any individual component. Many delude themselves that by just thinking, talking about or visualizing some component of the neigong, it will become established in their bodies—it will not.

Each component has general and specific considerations regarding how it is applied and incorporated into each of the different exercises. These considerations vary depending on whether you are standing still, moving, sitting, lying down or engaging in human interactions. Each component is taught separately and progressively and then is carefully integrated into each movement.

Generally, the components of neigong are not casually taught, especially for beginning and intermediate students. These techniques should be learned from a skilled instructor and the student's practice should be monitored and guided carefully.

One of the reasons that neigong was kept secret from the public for so long was that teachers did not want unnecessary problems (see Appendix C) to happen as a result of amateurs (whether students or teachers) misunderstanding the techniques or applying them incorrectly.

Each component must be thoroughly learned before going on to the next. This is not unlike learning advanced stages of music or opera—some stages can take years to be fully assimilated.

The danger with incomplete learning is that you can become unbalanced. The job of your instructor is to make sure that you do not.

Instructors must do their best to make sure:

- Students' energy remains smooth and does not become hyperactive.
- Students avoid dangerous practices.
- Students avoid addiction to over-stimulation.
- Students abide by the 70 percent rule.
- Students maintain clarity of mind.

Directly and Indirectly Experiencing Chi

The awareness of chi and the talent to be able to use it are forms of knowledge. Almost all students want to know how long will it take to understand chi and it is difficult to give an exact answer to this question. To paraphrase Confucius—some are born with knowledge, some obtain it through unremitting hard work, while others steal it or get it tangentially through an unpredictable side door.

Chi can be understood indirectly or directly. When your knowledge is indirect, you understand it through the sensations and effects it produces in your body and mind. When your knowledge is direct, you experience or feel chi as a distinct, tangible, living and concrete force.

At first, you will encounter chi only indirectly. However, over time, the possibility exists for you to experience and work with chi directly. The two easiest and most reliable of the 16 neigong components to use to make the jump from indirectly to directly experiencing chi are the first (breathing) and the seventh (opening and closing). The remaining neigong components are harder access routes to experiencing chi directly and as such are discussed only briefly.

The Complexity of Neigong

This section provides some insight into the complexity of each component, with the exceptions of components 12 through 15, which go beyond the scope of this book. Once you are comfortable with the basics of whatever qigong system you are studying, a good teacher will then help you learn particular aspects of neigong to incorporate into your practice.

Most of the information provided here concerns the first neigong component, breathing, because it is the easiest initial access point from which to obtain success in experiencing chi. More information on neigong can be found in my other books. For example, my book on Dragon and Tiger Medical Qigong primarily deals with the fifth (acupuncture channels) and eighth (etheric body) neigong components.

Neigong 1   Breathing Methods from the Simple to the Complex

Breathing is an excellent tool to show you how to feel inside your body and make all your systems work better. In Chapter 5's Longevity Breathing techniques, you learned some of the simplest components of breathing. In neigong, breathing methods become more complex. Once learned, they can be incorporated into any internal energy practice.

In the beginning stages of Longevity Breathing, you train your breathing mechanism until every internal part of your body is consistently and powerfully engaged in the breathing. This phase requires effort and consistent practice. It involves learning to breathe with your belly and abdomen and to bring air all the way up your back to the top of your lungs.

In the intermediate phase of Longevity Breathing, you will learn more complex methods. You will focus on getting your breathing to become progressively longer, softer and more silent. As you do so, the tightness and constrictions in your breathing mechanisms will gradually loosen and begin to move effortlessly with large amounts of motion. One day, you will have strong, deep, quiet and effortless breathing rhythms that you do not have to think about.

You also learn reverse breathing where all parts of your body move in synchronized fashion with your inhales and exhales. You learn to breathe from your skin and use your breath to open, strengthen and stabilize your etheric body.

You will learn circular breathing using your upper lungs, spine and lower tantien and how to integrate your breathing with any qigong exercise, using the other components of neigong.

The goal is to be able to breathe chi in and out of any body part at will through conscious intent alone.

Lengthening the Breath—Three Stages

Stage 1 Over millennia, Taoists observed that a thirty second breath was the minimum an average person should be able to do if he or she wanted to breathe well under normal circumstances. Yet given today's low standards where having a weak, shallow breath is considered normal, being able to easily do a thirty second breath may sound difficult to achieve. However since you will do countless millions of breaths from this day forward in your life, meeting this challenge will immeasurably better your life.

Stage 2 Taoists also observed that the body made a positive and profound life-altering shift when practitioners could extend their breath to two minutes. This causes major changes in the body and positively resets many of the body's energetic baselines. For example, the circulatory and nervous systems shift to another level of capability, which most people don't even know exists. Even if this ability is maintained only for a year, it usually causes a beneficial effect that lasts for decades. This ability can allow the practitioner to regularly shrug off stress that would otherwise be overwhelming and cause misery and poor health.

Stage 3 China was a nation that historically revered the wisdom old people could accumulate and consequently were greatly concerned with promoting longevity. China's Taoists were renowned for their longevity practices. An essential component of their most successful longevity techniques was turtle breathing. Giant turtles were known to live for hundreds of years. These turtles were commonly known to submerge and hold their breath for more than five minutes at a time. The turtle breathing aspect of Taoist breathing has the goal of generating five to eight minute breaths. This practice was known for its unsurpassed ability to transform and maintain an aged body and mind.

Connecting the Diaphragm, Belly and Internal Organs

Soft, springy ligaments connect your diaphragm to your internal organs and help them function and move the way nature designed them. For example, if your muscles are flaccid where ligaments connect to your liver, both the ligaments and the liver itself will have progressively poorer movement or even get stuck and barely move at all. This can, in a cascading effect, compromise the movements of your other organs.

Many of the fluid-pumping mechanisms of your body are connected to the movement of your diaphragm. Poor or unbalanced movement of your diaphragm compromises these flows. Strong rhythmic up and down diaphragmatic motions benefit and regularize these pumping actions.

Breathing with your belly strengthens your diaphragm. However, this must be learned systematically and gradually and should only be done with an instructor skilled in monitoring progressive stages. This is because the connections between your diaphragm and heart, if excessively forced, could get overstretched or dislodged.

There are specific exercises for making sure that your entire diaphragm muscle moves as a whole while exhaling and inhaling, without one part of the muscle being significantly stronger or weaker than another. Another set of exercises will teach you to lengthen the stretch of your diaphragm as you inhale and exhale.

Further exercises will teach you to feel your diaphragm clearly and evenly during breathing and to increase and release pressure gradually and evenly on your inhales and exhales.

This is important for the following reason. Just as breathing and chi are connected and directly influence each other, so are chi and blood. According to traditional Chinese medicine and qigong theory, chi, not just the physicality of the heart and vascular system, moves the blood. With practice, you can focus on your breathing to both sink your chi and consciously direct blood and chi to any part of your body.

Breathing into Your Lower Tantien

The object here is to wake up your lower tantien so you can feel it. This kind of breathing has progressive stages.

Stage one will teach you to have a very clear sense of breathing directly into your tantien, the energetic center of your body.

The next stage will teach you to feel whether the pressure of your belly expanding and contracting from your tantien might be unbalanced and, if so, how to balance it.

Practicing these exercises will expand your awareness so that you can notice all the minor variations of tension and contraction that occur as you breathe.

The next stage will teach you to breathe from your tantien in two or more directions simultaneously in several ways.

Reverse Breathing

In regular breathing, your belly expands as you inhale and shrinks when you exhale. In reverse breathing, you do the opposite—shrink your belly when you inhale and expand your belly when you exhale. Reverse breathing is sometimes called prebirth or womb breathing, because it is how babies breathe chi in and out of their bodies while in the womb.

The goals of reverse breathing include becoming aware of and controlling the subtle physical and energetic movements of your body so they deliberately occur in rhythm with your breathing. Every physical part and energetic function within your body and etheric body or aura will move in coordination with the expansions and contractions of your belly.

Reverse breathing opens, strengthens and stabilizes the aura and is integral to one aspect of what Lao Tse called "Breathing from the Heels," which, within Taoism, is considered to be the only truly complete breathing process.

Spinal Breathing

Spinal breathing opens and strengthens your spine and all the energies connected with it. Spinal breathing is taught in stages.

One stage involves energizing your spinal nerves and begins the process of connecting your spine's energy to your brain and upper tantien.

Another stage involves using your breath to move chi smoothly between your spine and the boundary of your etheric body.

Another stage will also teach you to smoothly and evenly move cerebrospinal fluid and energy within your spinal cord and up and down your spine.

Circular Breathing

Circular breathing is the smooth, seamless flow of chi through your nervous system during your inhales and exhales and most importantly during the change between them. It is an important quality of more advanced Taoist methods to link your breathing to physical movement and energy flow. Your breathing (inhales and exhales) should have no distinct starting or stopping points.

Circular breathing requires you to learn to mesh your breathing with your chi and nervous system so that they work together seamlessly.

Successful circular breathing requires that you accomplish five tasks:

1. Become aware of the underlying quality or feeling of your nervous system as you breathe.

2. Focus on the conjoined quality of your breath and nervous system as you inhale and exhale.

3. Find any gross gaps in your breathing, particularly at the changeover point between inhales and exhales.

4. Train your awareness to become increasingly subtle and conscious of the micro-gaps in your breathing. Make your breaths go progressively *sung* (p. 114). As this occurs, become aware of even more subtle gaps that cause your nervous system to freeze momentarily during your practice. You will train until your nervous system becomes completely smooth and seamless and the difference between inhales and exhales disappears.

5. The goal in the last phase of circular breathing is to directly find your chi. Having your breath be seamless and smooth can be the doorway to finding your chi; just as finding your chi is the doorway that can enable your breathing to become truly circular. They are interconnected and cannot be separated.

The task now is to make the jump from being only indirectly aware of your chi by its reflections in your breathing, nervous system and body (the goal of all previous text in this book), to becoming directly aware of chi as a separately-felt entity that empowers all movements in all your systems.

Awareness of subtleties and intentionality is a wonderful tool. As it becomes stronger and more refined it allows you to recognize and direct your energy in ways that otherwise would be impossible.

As you practice more and your breathing becomes seamless, the barriers to being aware of chi dissipate. Gradually, with more and more breathing practice, your awareness will learn to fully penetrate your nervous system and become exceedingly familiar with it. When this happens the last barriers to your breathing being fully circular will disappear.

Eventually, your awareness will be able to recognize the underlying separate qualities of your breathing, nervous system and chi. You will become aware of the subtle current which interlinks all three. You will experience how your chi affects, is affected by and is the underlying force that joins and controls your nervous system and breathing.

One day, as you focus on your breathing, the air coming in and out of your nose will seem to slow and then stop, while the insides of your abdomen and lungs will continue to move very powerfully. Even though you will be physically breathing well, it will seem as though your physical breath has gone totally silent and completely stopped and your body and mind have also spontaneously become silent.

An eerie silence and sense of incredibly expanded and empty space will arise within your body and mind. Suddenly you will find yourself silently breathing chi in and out.

Then, this too will seem to slow to a stop. One day, during the circular breathing process your body and mind spontaneously will again become even more silent. Even though you will be physically breathing well, it will seem as though your breath has gone totally silent and completely stopped.

Within this space your sense of air movement will be gone but your organs will restart opening and closing (expanding and condensing) as though they have an independent will of their own. Now, instead of air being moved in and out of your nose, each expanding and condensing of your internal organs will bring in and expel something. This is chi.

After becoming experienced with this for a while, you will have gained the foundation to gradually become able to directly move chi anywhere in your body by conscious intent alone, using all the components of neigong.

Neigong and Circularity

Let us return to the circular nature of the 16 neigong components:

- During your first revolution around the neigong circle you will indirectly experience and work with your chi.
- In the second revolution of the neigong circle, which can only begin after circular breathing has been accomplished, you can work directly with chi. You will practice the 16 neigong components to a dramatically greater depth, until your intent and manifestation of chi become precise and exceedingly adept.
- In the third revolution, you will move beyond qigong and into the realm of meditation. In Taoist thought, chi determines how well people function and achieve their potential. There is also what is called in Chinese the *yuan chi*, the universal energy that creates and moves the giant structures of the universe—galaxies, stars, planets, etc. In the third revolution of the neigong circle your task will be to become aware of and work with this universal consciousness. This is the path of the Tao.

Neigong 2 Moving Energy

There are many methods to help you feel your chi, so that you can move it smoothly to where it will be most useful and work most efficiently. Some of these methods are concerned with how to transform, dissolve and release the energy in specific ways within particular channels.

One technique will teach you to send chi smoothly down one side of your body and back up, on either the same or the opposite side.

Other techniques will teach you to move chi horizontally around your torso and activate your collateral acupuncture meridians, including the most important one called the *dai mai*.

Another technique, called wrapping, activates all your collateral meridians by moving chi through the connective tissues between the front of your torso and your spine.

Neigong 3 Alignments

The subject of precise body alignments becomes progressively more subtle and complex. In Chapter 9, you learned the fundamental alignments for the standing posture. The next stages will teach you to become progressively aware of and control specific alignments, their connections to other alignments and their physical, emotional and mental effects.

These physical alignments are extremely precise. They occur in all parts of your body and are often not intuitive. All create necessary space around your physical structures and help prevent them from collapsing or becoming too tightly compressed or overly loose.

Super-alignments exist in various kinds of balanced matched pairs, where each causes an opposite rising or falling pressure and chi movement in your body. There are also some complex and very subtle internal alignments that occur within your abdominal cavity.

There are also ways to align your chi in a coordinated manner within your energy channels, points and centers and your etheric field, as well as with your emotions and thoughts. In Taoist meditation, alignments go further and affect your psychic and karmic realms.

The specific techniques you will learn include:
- How to open the backs of your knee joints and your ankle joints.
- How to create more space inside your midriff.
- Precise ways to hold your head to cause specific effects in your mind
  and emotions.

- Alignments to control the movement of blood through your blood vessels.
- The exact way to align your tailbone, sacrum, spine and hips and how small movements in these alignments affect energy flow.
- Procedures for opening the kwa and shoulder's nest on each side of your body. This involves connecting them both physically and energetically so that you can move your internal organs to their optimum positions and maximize their functioning, blood flow and the energy within them.

Neigong 4 Dissolving

Advanced techniques for the outer or external dissolving process will teach you specific adaptations that can be used to dissolve chi anywhere, not only within yourself but potentially within another human being. Other techniques will show you how to dissolve blockages in your etheric body. Still others will teach you how to dissolve upward, towards and away from your lower tantien and simultaneously in multiple directions.

The inner dissolving process of Taoist meditation seeks to do the same for an individual's emotions, thoughts, psychic perceptions and karma.

Neigong 5 Main and Secondary Acupuncture Channels

Your acupuncture channels are your twelve main and eight extraordinary acupuncture meridians (secondary channels) and your 700-plus acupuncture points (see p. 254). These channels are located in your *wei chi*, which is a layer of chi located in the subcutaneous tissue found between your skin and muscles.

In this component of neigong, you will learn to become aware of and move energy through each acupuncture channel and connect it to others; how to activate particular acupuncture points; how to absorb and release energy through each channel and point; and how to vibrate energy at various acupuncture channels and points in various postures.

More advanced stages will teach you to feel and control the connections between your acupuncture channels, the right, left and central energy channels and the energies of your etheric body.

Neigong 6   Bending and Stretching

Stretching involves attempts to lengthen your muscle fibers and connective tissues either along the length of the muscles or, in more sophisticated techniques, at their insertion points, where muscles, ligaments and tendons attach to each other. In Taoist energy work, merely stretching your muscles is of secondary importance. The most important aspects of bending and stretching involve moving your soft tissues and fasciae in the direction of how you want energy to flow in your acupuncture meridians. This component will activate your yin and yang meridian flows by getting all the tissues below your skin to move in specific directions.

When this induced flow occurs you will be able to feel the sensation of movement under your skin.

In Western exercise, the stretching of muscles in one direction causes contraction in other muscles. In neigong, movements in one direction cause passivity rather than muscular contraction in the opposite direction. If you activate the movement of energy along a particular acupuncture meridian or energy channel, the muscles and tissue will move in that direction only. Once you learn to initiate movements in your body in a single direction only with your energy, muscular contraction or tension will not be required to do the physical movements of qigong and tai chi.

Neigong 7   Opening and Closing

Opening and closing actions (pulsing) occur in every part of your physical body, energy channels and etheric body.

Opening means to expand, grow larger, or flow outward and emanate. Closing means to gather in and, in most cases, get smaller. Closing carries no connotation of tension, contraction, collapsing or force in the movement, only continuous inward flow toward a point of origination.

Specific techniques will be taught to empower you to open and close the spaces within your joints and spine and inside and between your internal organs, all bodily fluids, energy points, channels and centers within your body and in the energy fields connected to you.

In this part of the neigong system, you will be taught to become aware of and then deliberately open and close every body part that has the potential to move. This opening and closing is essential and lies at the root of understanding within the physical body how yin and yang functions and how to directly experience your chi. This is ultimately responsible for the changing functions of yin and yang both within yourself and the universe.

Opening and closing methods may be practiced independently or done in a whole-body, integrated fashion with either regular or reverse breathing.

Neigong 8 The Etheric Body or Aura

The energy of your etheric body or aura connects with the energies of your body and mind and with the psychic and spiritual forces that exist in the universe. First, you will be taught to become aware of and control these connections inside yourself, then to become aware of the energies in the universe, and finally to learn to use your energies so you can move in harmony with the universe. If you wish to absorb and use the power of the universe, you first have to learn to make your own energies harmonious with it.

Neigong 9 Spiraling

This component is about becoming aware of, controlling and amplifying the circles and spirals of chi in your body.

Physical techniques include:

- Circular and spiraling physical movements.
- Twisting your soft tissues.
- Inward or outward curving of muscles at critical junctures of your body.
- Spiraling your soft tissues.

Energetic techniques include:

- Using awareness and intention to create circles, spheres and spirals of energy within your body and outside of it.
- Becoming sensitive to and using energetic spirals.
- Emitting spiraling chi from your lower tantien and connecting it through specific pathways to anywhere in your body.

Neigong 10 Absorbing and Projecting

Learning to absorb and project chi to or from anywhere inside or outside your body at will is central to qigong self-healing capabilities, hands-on and psychic healing, meditation and internal martial arts.

Stages of learning this component include:

- Absorbing and projecting chi from your three tantiens.
- Learning to clearly master intentionality.
- Quieting your mind so that it can be aware of the totality of what it means to absorb and project chi under different circumstances.

Neigong 11 The Spine

Many techniques exist for awakening and controlling all the energies of your spinal system and its connections to your three tantiens. Your spinal system includes your vertebrae, cerebrospinal fluid and spinal cord. These techniques make it possible for you to heal back and neck problems and potentially regenerate spinal discs.

The Taoist Spine Stretch taught in this book is a preliminary exercise of this component of this neigong component. Other techniques will teach you to precisely control the movements of: 1) each vertebra in all directions independently of muscular movement; 2) cerebrospinal fluid; and 3) the plates of your skull. Other techniques will teach you to do internal pumping to increase, decrease and otherwise manipulate the spaces between your vertebrae, which can relieve or cure problems related to slipped or degenerating discs.

More advanced techniques will teach you to work directly with the energies that run through the various layers of your spinal cord.

Neigong 12–15 The Left, Right and Central Channels and Three Tantiens

The Taoist perspective holds that to genuinely learn and activate neigong components 12 through 15, the practitioner must have a solid foundation in the more sophisticated aspects of the first 11 neigong components and be able to integrate these components together seamlessly. Only after this is achieved can all the neigong components genuinely link and become coordinated with your right, left and central energy channels and three tantiens (*Figures 15-2* and *15-3*) and thereby allow neigong to fully manifest its potential power.

Neigong 16 Integration

All the components of the neigong system must integrate with each other in your practice until they result in a single, unified energy. The goal of integration is to effortlessly use neigong to empower all aspects of your life.

It is useful to recognize that merely being able to create temporary energetic states or experiences is different from stabilizing energy within you.

All the components of neigong are useful for martial arts, meditation and healing yourself and others.

Qigong Is the Foundation for Shengong

In China, the esoteric side of qigong/neigong is *shengong*, which means spirit power. *Shen* means spirit, *gong* means the power or the practice that enables you to do something.

Shengong is said to develop psychic and mystical powers, such as clairvoyance, the ability to walk through walls, walk on water and raise the dead, etc.

Many religious practices have esoteric traditions that are surrounded by stories and mythology about what their practitioners can do. India and Tibet refer to psychic powers as *siddhi*, the fruits of accomplishment, whereas in China they are called *te i gong neng*, special abilities gained through practice. In India's yogic tradition, psychic powers are developed through pranayama, mantras and working with chakras; in Tibet through *sa lung* (wind and channels) and *tumo* (the yoga of inner fire); and in Taoism with shengong.

All the Eastern traditions hold that these powers or gifts of the spirit are intrinsic to humans but can only be accessed, developed and actualized through deep spiritual practice.

Incorporating neigong into qigong or other Taoist energy practices provides the foundation that can lead to the study of shen gung, but only if and when a practitioner convinces an authentic teacher that he or she is ready.

These esoteric practices, whatever the tradition, are seldom talked about or casually taught. Their existence can be a somewhat contentious issue and may be hotly debated. Shengong is classically considered to be a part of the higher-level teachings of neigong.

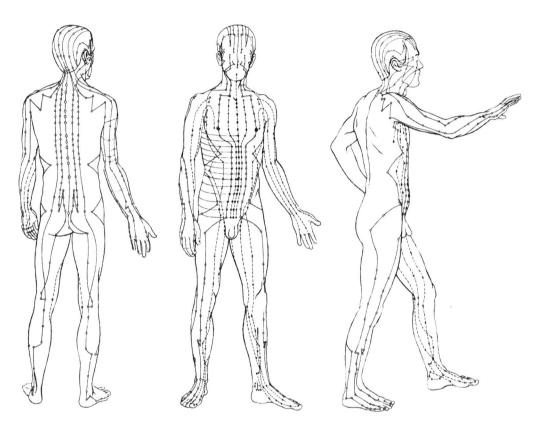

The acupuncture meridian lines of the body and points along them through which chi circulates.

Figure 15-4

Afterword

An Abundance of Chi Is Your Birthright

People in the Orient have developed methods that allow a human being to have tremendous vitality well past the point that the body is naturally overflowing with energy. Many of the practices developed in China have been kept secret for centuries, but I believe that now it is time for all human beings to have the chance to benefit from this profound life-serving knowledge.

From the ancient Taoist point of view, the vast majority of human beings are given plenty of energy at birth. At some point, though, if one has not lived a completely natural and healthy life (which is getting progressively more difficult all the time) this energetic abundance begins to fade, and more energy must be earned. A young blade of grass, a seedling tree and a baby are soft and flexible. With the coming of old age, the blade of grass hardens and can be easily snapped; the tree becomes brittle and dry; and elderly human beings stiffen until they can barely move.

You Must Practice to Reap the Benefits

Abundant life energy, the ancient Taoists observed, came with softness and pliability. The core qigong exercises in this book provide the foundation necessary to regain these qualities, but this path does require time and effort. While the intellectual information in this book may be interesting in itself, the real value of this book can only come through the practice of these exercises. The proof is in eating the pudding, not in reading about what it tastes like.

Those who are thinking of learning tai chi chuan or any internal martial art will find that learning and practicing these core qigong exercises will increase their learning speed dramatically. I have personally seen in the United States and Europe many people who have practiced tai chi chuan for ten or fifteen years and yet are not familiar with the basic principles these core exercises involve—principles, which in authentic tai chi, they should have been exposed to in their first year of practice. If anyone is thinking of learning tai chi or the internal martial arts, this is the best foundation possible.

For average people, who do not want to get into the complicated movements of tai chi but would like to gain a significant number of the mental and physical benefits available from tai chi, the *Opening the Energy Gates of Your Body* exercises are perfect. Later, if these benefits really inspire those people to learn tai chi, hsing-i, or bagua, they will already have the best possible foundation and will be far ahead of most beginners.

APPENDIX A:

Guidelines for Practice

Practice Until Your Joints Feel Well-Lubricated

Often, individuals will reach a point in standing where they feel they have had enough— the body wants to move. At this point, begin Cloud Hands. Continue Cloud Hands until the contraction and stiffness of the body begins to go away and the major areas of immobility loosen up. This activity can be thought of as the dry areas inside the body becoming wet and lubricated, especially your joints, hips, spine, and waist. When the body begins to feel oiled, go on to the First Swing. Repeat this process through each of the swings: when "oiled" by one swing, proceed on to the next. After becoming proficient in these exercises, most people find that three to five minutes of Cloud Hands and one to two minutes of the swings is enough. Up to a point, the more time spent on each swing, the more lubricated the joints will become.

If You Feel Pain, Use Slower and Smaller Movements

If for some reason pain comes up as a result of overstrain, simply go on to the next swing, or, if the pain is severe, back off, rest and assess whether it is time to stop practicing for the day. The primary rule in these exercises is to do no harm to your body.

A distinction must be made between the natural strain of exercise or stretching and the pain of damage. Pain in any of the joints means you should back off immediately and review the instructions on how to do the exercise. If the instructions are being followed correctly and you get pain in a joint—whether elbow, knee, shoulder, or wrist—you could be overstraining yourself or opening up an old injury. In either case, moderate the range and pace of your movements, and if the pain continues beyond the mild stage, switch into the next swing. If it persists into the next swing, decrease your range of motion until the pain stops. Under no circumstances should you attempt to "work through" pain in your joints. This same rule applies when you practice tai chi chuan, hsing-i, or bagua, or, for that matter, any internal exercise.

The soft tissue of the body is another matter. The small motions of qigong may lead to burning or knifelike feelings in the soft tissue. The School of Hard Knocks invariably teaches most people what is meant by overdoing it in this regard. If the pain is severe, unless you are under the guidance of a master, back off. All athletes must learn to recognize their limits, and if you do not have much experience, it is best to err on the side of caution. Slight pain in the soft tissue is quite normal; a lot of pain is best avoided.

Most people do not know their limits, and consequently overdo it. This is particularly true of weekend athletes. While overdoing for a few seconds will not cause much damage, really pushing it for longer periods of time and over many days certainly will. Of course, the amount of strain a given individual can bear depends on many factors, such as age, weight, body type, and previous training.

Special Warning: Do Not Overstrain Knee Joints

Overstraining muscles will at worst result in a pull; the vast majority of people will stop well before that stage due to the pain involved. A pulled or overstrained muscle will heal within a few days, a few weeks, or, at worst, in a few months. On the other hand, tendon, ligament, or joint damage can last a lifetime and even require surgery. Be gentle with your joints—they are not replaceable. Muscles grow back, but joints do not.

For most people, pain in the knees or ankles means they need to stand a little higher. I really want to caution Westerners in general that they live in an upper-body culture, accompanied by poor awareness of the joints in the lower body. In martial arts, this lack of awareness all too commonly leads to knee problems. The internal martial arts are known in China for their ability to heal back and joint problems. If you strain your joints, however, the twisting actions can easily weaken already weak structures and aggravate old injuries. These exercises can be of tremendous benefit if done correctly, but, like any type of exercise, they can also damage people who try to be heroes and go beyond their limits.

Movement Artists: If You Feel Fatigue, Change to the Next Swing

People involved in movement arts will usually only be satisfied with the greatest possible range of movement. This desire will cause them to want to go beyond getting the joints lubricated to a sense of the joints dissolving and even a feeling of bonelessness. When this feeling is achieved, you are ready to switch to the next exercise. This is very difficult to put in terms of time, as it is possible to do Cloud Hands or each of the swings as much an hour (or two, or three) at a time. This is very individual, and only in a face-to-face encounter with a highly skilled instructor can exact parameters be stated. As a general rule, however, if fatigue begins to set in at one of the joints, it is time to move on to the next exercise. The trick is to optimize the amount of energy running through the system, without going over the line of exhaustion. This can only be done through self-observation, which leads to the direct understanding and experience of the limits as well as the strengths and possibilities of your body and mind.

Martial Artists: Do Not Visualize Fighting Applications

For the martial artist, the previously discussed exhaustion and joint strain issues also apply. Additionally, martial artists tend to visualize all sorts of fighting applications, as these are inherent in the exercises. The tendency is to get so wrapped up in martial arts applications that the body's limits are forgotten, either intentionally or unintentionally. Try to avoid this mistake, for as well as damaging the joints it can create mental tension around the fighting techniques.

Best Time to Practice

The optimum times to practice may not be realistic for most people. As with most energy development exercises, the best time to practice begins about two hours before dawn, which is when the earth is most quiet and psychic disturbance is lowest. Another good time is early in the morning, around sunrise. Practice in the morning is best on an empty stomach, so that the energy of the body is not being dissipated by digesting breakfast. Have breakfast afterwards.

Early evening is also a good time, though one should avoid exercising too close to bedtime, as these practices generate energy. If you do practice before going to bed, do the First Swing, then the Spine Stretch, then the First Swing again, this time doing it so that you actually feel as if you are falling asleep on your feet—let all your remaining tension fall into the ground. For night owls, the period between midnight and 3 A.M. is quite favorable for practicing as the stresses and psychic disturbances generated by city life have begun to wind down. During these hours, the body is also naturally beginning to fill up with yang chi, and practicing qigong will accelerate this process. Night owls normally lose yang chi by not sleeping during these hours; the practice of qigong during these hours mitigates this problem. This is the perfect practice time for people who work the swing shift.

Bear in mind that the best time to practice is anytime, rather than not at all.

How Often Should I Practice?

1. General public: a minimum of three to five times a week

The first question on people's lips usually has to do with how much or how often to practice these exercises. For the first three years, it is strongly recommended to practice these exercises for a minimum of 10 to 20 minutes per session at least three or four times a week. Daily is best.

2. Martial artists: daily

If you are practicing tai chi chuan or other internal martial arts, after about three years you will have the sensitivity to work out your own practice session, but ideally these exercises should be done every day. Use all the Energy Gates exercises as a warm-up before your main workout, and use the swings and the Spine Stretch as an excellent wind down. Employed for these purposes, the swings only need to be done for two or three minutes.

3. Runners and athletes: warm up and cool down

People involved in activities such as running or competitive sports will find that the swings and the Spine Stretch are excellent ways to release the stress and chi blockage that can occur after competition. These exercises will improve your recovery time dramatically. They help loosen and lubricate the body prior to activity.

4. Office workers: lunch and short breaks

It is exceedingly useful for people in high stress jobs to do the swings and Spine Stretch for a few minutes during coffee breaks, when they are first feeling stressed, but before the stress has had a chance to settle in. A minute spent getting rid of stress at this stage can be incredibly valuable. The swings are recommended when there is only a minute or two to do something.

Use Qigong to Manage Stress

For people involved in high-stress jobs, it is important to understand how stress works. Stress begins with overexcitement of the nervous system and then slowly works its way deep into the body. It begins as wet cement, so to speak, and when the stress is prolonged this begins to harden (i.e., the contraction and constriction of the nerves and organs starts to become permanent). The stress of the morning begins to harden around lunch time. The stress accumulated after lunch will begin to set by evening or the end of the work day.

Five minutes spent doing the swings or Cloud Hands during a coffee break in the morning or the afternoon can prove to be of great value, in effect wiping away the day's stress and keeping the metaphorical cement wet. Ten or fifteen minutes at lunch can bring back the freshness of the morning. Practice after work can take away all the stress ("wet cement") accumulated during the day.

So far we have only discussed getting rid of the stress accumulated during the day. Any practice above and beyond this initial stress release will increase your core energy reserves, which your body and mind uses in times of crisis, emergency, or recovery from illness or accident. This core reserve of chi will also determine the quality of energy available later in your life.

Toxin Release Will Be Followed by Energy Flow

It needs to be kept in mind that in the early stages of practice (the first few months), these exercises may cause the body to release a tremendous amount of stored toxins, which can result in feelings of fatigue, discomfort, and an unwillingness to practice. Toxins are released through the sweat, urine, and feces, and in the beginning you may notice that your sweat smells unpleasant. This will pass, and soon your sweat will be relatively odorless.

While not a substitute for fasting and other cleansing methods, the core qigong exercises in this book, and the internal martial arts in general, are good additional cleansing therapies. Once the initial layers of toxins and trapped energy are released, the energizing effects of these exercises will begin to be felt twenty-four hours a day.

Special Note for Women

Qigong causes increases blood circulation. Thus, during the menstrual cycle, there is a possibility that qigong practice may cause excessive menstrual bleeding. The Chinese medical view is that if your menstrual bleeding is in fact increased during qigong practice, you should reduce your practice time or cease practicing altogether until your period is over.

Special Note for Men

Unless you have learned to regulate the internal flow of your chi during sexual intercourse and control your ejaculations, it is best to avoid practicing qigong two to three hours before and after intercourse. This avoids unbalancing the regulated flow of chi gained through qigong practice and prevents excessive energy loss.

APPENDIX B:
Searching for a Qualified Teacher

It is considerably easier to find a good qigong instructor than a genuine neigong teacher. Not only are there far more people who teach qigong rather than neigong, but also it is more difficult to be accepted as a student of a neigong teacher, particularly if you do not have much experience in neigong.

Finding a Qigong Teacher

Instructions in qigong must be followed accurately, and especially in the early stages of learning, it is important to have access to a competent teacher, so that in the small number of cases where problems arise, help is not far away. The instructions given in this book about chi movement, rather than body mechanics, are not meant to be learned solely from the printed word. These instructions are meant to enhance understanding while one is under the guidance of a qualified instructor.

The teacher needs to demonstrate to the student verbally, nonverbally, and by the quality of his life, what it is that the student is trying to do. If the teacher's chi is not full, if the teacher is not essentially relaxed, then it is highly unlikely that the student's chi will become full and relaxed. Qigong is not the acquisition of intellectual information, but is the process of becoming something. The person you model yourself after will also be imparting his or her energy to you. The quality of that person's energy will determine what you will get from the interaction. In China it is put very simply: this kind of subject can only be learned from somebody who has got it. Many forms of athletic or intellectual skill can be learned from a good coach who is a poor practitioner. However, in chi development, the level of the teacher's accomplishment determines his capacity to transmit this development to the student. Ideal teachers are those whose personal chi is highly developed, as is their capacity to communicate to the student. As the old saying goes, "Some people can teach, some people can do, and those who can do both are very rare."

Do not be misled by a good pitch, for the words of chi development are much easier to talk about than do. Also, be aware that an Oriental ethnic origin is no guarantee of expertise. Take your time, and check out all the teachers in your area (if there are any).

Only learn qigong from someone you sense is on the up and up. It might be better to wait than to get involved in studying qigong with somebody you are unsure of.

In the United States and Europe, at this moment, only a minority of the instructors would be considered competent by generally recognized traditional standards in China—standards that have been established over thousands of years of consistent experimentation and bitter experience. Though these traditional standards commonly do not guarantee fast and easy results, they generally allow students to reach their goals with sufficient effort and practice.

What to Look for in a Good Teacher

When considering qigong teachers, the first questions to ask are: Have they been doing the type of chi work they are asking you to do for a minimum of ten years? Did they really understand their teacher's transmission, especially if their teacher did not speak the same language? Do they seem fairly well balanced psychologically? If they are essentially open-minded, open-hearted, and generous of spirit, then you have a much better chance of getting the story straight. If they are not, and use information as a carrot to entice you, their neuroses may keep them from giving out the real stuff. Look for mental and emotional clarity and physical well-being in a teacher.

Unfortunately, even if they do meet the above criteria, they may not know enough to debug their system if something goes wrong. Look for brutally honest and scrupulous teachers who have studied many systems completely and understand how they interface, or at the very least, know their own system down to the finest details. Then, if problems do occur, they are likely to be competent and willing to work with you to overcome your difficulties. Many Chinese learned as youngsters and teach adults, not realizing that the process of learning is different for children than adults.

Talk to ongoing students of a particular teacher to get a picture of what their practice is like—find out if they are getting something you would like to have. As the years pass, more and more Americans will be able to discriminate between good and bad qigong, and you will be able to consult with them about what is going on.

Finding a Neigong Teacher

I have been working with chi since the 1960s, including over a decade of training in China. I found that determining whether a teacher was qualified to teach neigong was neither clear-cut nor simple. Good, authentic teachers are hard to find, particularly in the West, but worth seeking out, even if you have to travel far to find them. A teacher that embodies some or all of the neigong system will have as much or more relevant training and experience as any Ph.D. would have in his or her particular field.

Although China has a system for ranking teachers of Taoist energy practices, none exists in the West. This is one reason why the transference of the subtle knowledge of neigong to the West is so difficult.

In order to find teacher appropriate for your level of learning, whether in the West or in China, here are some points to consider:

- Teachers that have some knowledge of a few components of neigong are more plentiful than teachers with higher-level knowledge. These teachers may be able to teach you the foundational material that inspires you to seek out higher level teachers.
- Teachers of qigong and tai chi may know and teach little, some or all of the 16 neigong components. You cannot judge how much a teacher knows by his or her ethnicity or by whether or not there is fame, marketing cachet or a title attached to his or her name.
- Safe, but not always guaranteed, are older and perhaps "famous" masters whose skill and value to students has been proven by the test of time and reputation. This is especially true of those that hold very old, established lineages.
- Genuinely knowledgeable neigong masters may not like to fully and openly teach neigong and may not be easily convinced to do so or to take on a new student.
- A teacher who knows how to apply neigong within one context of using chi— such as self healing, personal health maintenance, healing others, martial arts or meditation—may or may not know how to apply the neigong to other contexts or even have any training in their application.
- Language barriers between Chinese and your language may need to be overcome.
- People who have spent years in the field investigating who's who can point you in the right direction. Better yet, find someone who may be able to intercede with a reputable teacher so that they will accept rather than reject you.
- The personalities of neigong teachers and masters run the gamut from friendly to abrasive, humble to arrogant. Do not let what you perceive as a teacher's negative personality traits get in the way of learning from someone with genuine and authentic knowledge.

APPENDIX C:

Importance of Correct Qigong Practice

The vast majority of the thousands of qigong techniques, including those found in this book, are health-enhancing and safe. However, like any powerful tool, if used incorrectly, qigong can cause damage as well as benefit. There are literally hundreds of qigong practices that can cause significant problems, and it would be impossible to mention every one. Here I will endeavor to give the reader a healthy respect for the power of qigong techniques and some means to discern which techniques are safe and effective.

Every Body Is Different

Humans have different levels of tolerance to stress and pressure. Some lead completely dissolute lifestyles and live long, healthy lives, while others live as purely as possible and have short, miserable lives. The difference lies mainly in the amount of energy they were born with and the strength of their nervous systems.

From the Chinese point of view, the capacity to bear stress is a function of the strength of the nerves. When the stress level surpasses the central nervous system's capacity to handle it, the nerves begin to break down, which results in all sorts of physical, emotional, and mental disturbances, and can eventually lead to organ malfunction and premature death.

Chi Travels through the Nerves

Since different people have nervous systems of different strengths, it is important that practices take this difference into account. Just as a lifestyle that some thrive on would send others to an early grave, so some qigong systems that are fine for some are actually quite dangerous for others.

Chi travels through the nerves, and consequently it is the nerves that are potentially most at risk from incorrect qigong practice. While proper qigong practice strengthens the nerves, improper techniques can overload them and lead to the breakdown of all body systems.

Every message from the brain to the body, and vice versa, goes through the central nervous system. When practicing direct manipulation of the central nervous system, three precautions must be taken: 1) Practice must be done within the proper limits, or the nerves will be damaged; 2) New pathways must lead to health and well-being, not towards illness; and 3) The body must have enough time to balance out all these new inputs, so that the signal does not get scrambled. Going too fast can cause serious problems for both the mind and body, as well as lead to hallucinations (imagining things are happening when they are not).

It has been proven consistently in China that qigong, if practiced correctly, can bring about a reversal of internal organ malfunctions and can relieve all manner of stress by increasing the strength of the nerves. If done incorrectly, however, it can instead actually increase stress or damage organs, just as a mechanic, using the same tools, can damage a car as easily as fix it.

Safety Comparison of Pranayama and Qigong

"Prana" in Sanskrit and "chi" in Chinese can both be translated as "the breath of life." The classic yoga texts, when discussing pranayama (energy development), always state that the most important requirement for learning is the guidance of a competent teacher on a frequent, preferably daily basis. This requirement is based on the following presuppositions:

- Pranayama is inherently dangerous.
- To avoid pitfalls, it must be practiced correctly.
- If for some reason problems arise, the teacher must be on the spot to correct them before it is too late.
- Signs too subtle for a novice to notice will arise before problems develop. Slight calibrations at this stage can mean the difference between learning correctly and self-injury.

Pranayama Is Based on Breathing and Packing

Pranayama utilizes techniques that close down energy in one part of the body and build it up (pack it) in another. These techniques involve postures and the use of the breath.

As such, pranayama is an extremely precise science. Just as in a nuclear reactor it is crucial to develop exactly the correct amount of heat and pressure, so it is in pranayama— and on an individual level the consequences of incorrect practice can be devastating.

In the West, as well as India, many people who practice pranayama techniques incorrectly suffer from physical and psychic problems as a result. Much of this is simply the result of a lack of competence on the part of the teacher, though it also can come from a frivolous disregard for what the teacher taught. In America, especially, there are those who learn only from books. Such people do not have any way to be aware of potential problems, to know how much is enough, and to recognize what practices require the guidance of a teacher.

The difficulty with pranayama practices lies not in the fact that they do not work, but rather that they work too well. If a technique has power, its power to benefit life is sometimes matched by its power to destroy it when practiced incorrectly or by a person of the wrong constitution.

Benefit-to-Risk Relationship in Qigong

In hatha yoga pranayama, which have the ability to initiate and carry through the genuine kundalini process to self-realization, the potential benefits are roughly equivalent to the potential risks. In qigong however, the relationship between risk and benefit is more complex—some systems have low benefits and high risks, some average amounts of each, and some, like the techniques discussed in this book, have very low risks and high benefits.

Learning Qigong in China

Even in China it is very difficult to find a good qigong teacher. Most teachers impart only one system, and teach that system as they learned it—by rote. They have no basic understanding of how it works and how it fits into the overall picture of qigong.

The Chinese make a great distinction between people who know some qigong techniques and people who are qigong masters. This distinction is much like that between a computer operator and a computer programmer. The former knows how to push the buttons to make the system work, but doesn't know what to do if something goes wrong, or how to modify the system for specific needs. On the other hand, the programmer, or computer master, knows how to get the "bugs" out of the system should they appear, and how to adjust the program for a specific application or a particular user.

Students rarely investigate different qigong systems before beginning to practice one, and once they have begun qigong with a given teacher, it is considered disloyal to even visit other teachers. Their teacher's word becomes gospel. This climate makes it hard for Chinese students to become expert in more than one branch of qigong.

Taoists Stress the Spiritual Framework of Qigong

China is the oldest continuously civilized culture on earth and the Chinese are incredibly proud of that fact. Historically, they have considered themselves the only civilized nation on earth. When this attitude is combined with the memory of how poorly Westerners have treated them in the past, it is understandable that many qigong masters do not want to have anything to do with foreigners, and are especially unwilling to give out one of the gems of Chinese civilization.

Though many Chinese martial arts masters would not teach me the real stuff or would teach me incorrectly, the Taoists were beyond cultural and personal differences. They found it admirable that a Westerner would take the time and trouble to learn their language to be able to study something (qigong) that they considered very important. The Taoists were generally highly developed spiritually, and considered the development of spiritual life to transcend time, space, and culture. The majority of in-depth qigong work I have learned was taught to me by this group, and without them it would have been impossible for me to make sense of this subject.

Comparing Qigong Systems

One thing I saw very clearly during the course of my studies was that many types of qigong consistently caused problems in a certain percentage of practitioners, while other types did not seem to do all that much either positively or negatively. I also saw that some systems had broad applications, so that the same techniques could be used to benefit many different problems, while some were very specific. Some systems mixed well with others, whereas some did not.

The following cases illustrate some of the difficulties that can arise from the improper practice of qigong. In each of these cases I have either known the individual personally or the problem has actually occurred to me. I was extremely lucky that my first teacher, Wang Shu Jin taught me only safe practices, but later on I learned a number of dangerous practices, some of which caused me great harm. Though I originally did not believe that qigong could cause problems, I found out the hard way that it could.

Improper Qigong Practice Can Cause Problems

In rare instances, qigong done improperly has the potential to make people ill or worsen their mental and physical health. The Chinese term for this is *dzuo huo lu mo* "fire goes to the devil."

Too Much Chi Is Painful

My teacher Liu Hung Chieh passed on his hsing-i and bagua lineage to only one other person, Bai Hua. Bai Hua at one time taught in Amoy (Xiamen, Fukien Province), and this case concerns one of his students.

Bai Hua taught this student the basic hsing-i neigong practice of sinking the chi to the lower tantien and after about two years of practice his student began to get very powerful. At this time Bai Hua left Amoy for another city, and his student began to visit a number of hsing-i masters, looking for secret techniques from each. What he learned he practiced diligently, knowing that his first technique had worked so well.

Unfortunately his perseverance backfired. After a year practicing these techniques, though none were inherently bad, the combination resulted in all sorts of problems. In his effort to build chi in his lower tantien he ended up forcing his chi below his tantien and into his genitals. He effectively emptied the chi from his middle burner (internal organs) into his lower burner. This breaking of the natural energetic seal between the middle and lower burners left his middle burner chi in total disarray. This resulted in mental and physical problems, including involuntary semen emissions and hallucinations. He lost his job, and his impending marriage had to be postponed indefinitely.

It took an herbal master and Bai Hua three years to bring him back to near normal. It takes much less time to do damage to your chi than to fix it. Imagine if this had happened in America—the chance of finding genuine experts capable of treating this student's problems would be slim indeed.

Sexual Qigong Can Be Dangerous

Many people today are fascinated by qigong techniques for developing sexual power. There is a system, for instance, that includes techniques such as forcibly sucking energy up the anus and spine and hanging weights of ever-increasing amounts from the testicles and penis.

Around 1970, Wang Shu Jin, my first teacher and a man known for his Taoist sexual abilities, warned me against this technique. Then, when I mentioned it to my next teacher, Hung I Hsiang, he told me that it would be a very bad idea for me to practice the technique. In fact, he gave me a one-hour lecture to caution me about practicing ridiculous forms of esoteric sexual qigong.

Lesser problems are even more common. I have met many people who have practiced sexual control techniques and damaged their sexual apparatus. It is easy to overstrain the system, especially if the sexual organs are genetically weak to begin with. Some common problems include swollen testicles and internal bleeding. While these practices may lead to the ability to maintain erections for a longer time, the increased pressure can damage the underlying tissues. Women, too, can be damaged by inappropriate sexual qigong practices, resulting in problems such as false pregnancies and erratic periods.

For men, another sexual qigong and martial arts practice that can cause problems involves sucking the testicles up into the body. In martial arts this technique is used to protect oneself from groin kicks. Wang Shu Jin advised me not to practice this technique because I was traveling too often, and he couldn't monitor me closely enough. He also said that, even with close monitoring a certain percentage of people are damaged by it, if the practice is begun after puberty.

Close supervision by a master is highly recommended when learning any sexual qigong practices. America is now a workshop culture, where material that was traditionally presented over months is presented in a day or two or even an hour.

In Taoism, it is traditional to avoid teaching potentially dangerous material without all possible precautions. In some traditions, it is felt that if the majority is helped and only a minority may be harmed, overall more good than harm is being done. It is important for students of such techniques to be aware that they could be one of this minority, and might not know about the dangers until too late.

I will only publicly teach qigong techniques that are virtually risk-free. Only privately, where I can provide proper supervision, will I teach riskier material that has potentially faster results than the very safe techniques. In a way, the difference is like putting your money in a money market account, where growth is slow, steady, and sure, or playing fast and loose with your money in the stock market or commodities.

The Downside of Packing Chi

Hung I Hsiang's brother was a practitioner of White Crane qigong. A common technique of Shaolin qigong methods such as White Crane is to force, or "pack," energy into the body, much like forcing clothes into a suitcase. This involves forceful breathing, body contractions, and a sense of physical and energetic strength. By overdoing it, Hung I Hsiang's brother actually caused one of his lungs to hemorrhage, and died.

In the West, I have seen people practicing all sorts of chi packing exercises, and these techniques are all potentially dangerous if not carefully supervised over time. Forceful packing can potentially cause internal hemorrhaging, imbalances in the overall body energy, damage to lung tissue and susceptibility to respiratory diseases.

A karate practitioner in her late forties came to see me in Boston, who because of practicing a packing exercise she had learned in a workshop, had suffered pneumonia for the last four winters. The practice she had learned was quite forceful. She had been perfectly healthy before. I found that she had been practicing diligently but incorrectly. After I worked with her, she went through the next winter without getting pneumonia. Fortunately, her case was correctable, but many are not.

Another person, an assistant instructor of a well-known East Coast martial arts master, was told to practice Small Heavenly (Microcosmic) Orbit in a forceful way, using reverse breathing to generate heat in the lower tantien, which was then circulated. This person was also told to squeeze his anus and forcibly lift energy up his spine with his breathing.

The more he did this, the stronger and more powerful his energy felt. As in other qigong techniques, the greater the force used, the stronger the experience generated. Unfortunately, he was burning himself up, especially his kidney and heart energy. When he began to experience symptoms such as cold, clammy sweats, involuntary tremors, extreme sensitivity to cold, and loss of vitality he was told to keep practicing, to "burn through the blockage." Even though he stopped these practices, it took more than five years of working on the problem to get rid of the symptoms.

The fact that these symptoms arose is not in itself dire, since they could have been corrected at an early stage. His teacher failed to pay attention to the warning signals and, instead, made the student feel that there was something wrong with him! If your body or mind experiences great difficulties when you practice qigong, simply stop. The trouble may not reside in you, but rather in faulty teaching or your misunderstanding of the instructions.

Vibrating Chi Can Have Unpleasant Side Effects

In many qigong systems, especially Shaolin style and animal styles (White Crane, for example) there is a technique that deliberately tries to vibrate chi in the body. The breath oscillates rapidly, and chi is vibrated inside bones, tissues, brain and so forth.

This type of practice may have a number of unpleasant side effects. It can make a person absolutely uncaring, and, as the vibrations get stronger, it can bring on a kind of megalomania, or other mental illnesses. It can also cause physical hallucinations, where sensations of shaking, opening and closing continue after practice has stopped. If these practices are continued long enough, they can cause problems in the internal organs. The lungs and liver are the most vulnerable, but other organs are susceptible as well.

It is quite common in these practices for the chi to be incompletely or irregularly circulated, rather than fully awakened and circulated. When I first saw these vibrating practices in Beijing, it was very obvious that the way they were forcing chi was causing what in India would be called irregularly awakened kundalini.

My medical qigong teacher in Beijing, Zhang Jia Hua, informed me that these types of vibratory practices historically had a high casualty rate. She had worked with cancer patients who had brought their symptoms under control with qigong and then begun vibratory practices, which brought their cancer out of remission, and they returned to the hospital to die. The strong sense of power makes these practices addictive, and like crack, when the crash comes, it is too late.

When I was 21 I was taught a "secret" technique. I was told it was the qigong that was the power behind tai chi. I practiced this technique diligently, two hours a day, until I was able to break bones with one slap simply by vibrating my energy. At the same time, I noticed an incredibly seductive feeling of energy in my head, and I began to realize I was becoming psychotic. The stronger this chi got, the stranger my mind became, and the hotter my body felt.

In a particularly raucous martial art incident in Japan, I found I was breaking bones left and right, and was almost unable to stop myself. At this point, I realized this practice was making me crazy, removing compassion from my makeup, and I stopped. When I returned to Taiwan a few years later, I found I had been practicing the Tsung He form of Fukien White Crane, and that some of the practitioners of this art were either subtly or obviously psychotic. Many of the most humble-seeming masters of this type of qigong were actually the most dangerous. Power replaced compassion, and while they might use their power for healing, it would be of little concern to them if they accidentally caused damage instead.

A student of tai chi in San Diego (let's call him Mike) studied with an instructor who taught a form that involved vibrating the mind, body, and breath. He was in his teens at the time, with no martial arts background, and thought this was traditional tai chi chuan. His first year felt good and relaxed, but then his teacher wanted to increase his pace. Weapon forms and more breathing practices were added to increase the vibration. About two-and-a-half years into his training, he developed the ability to discharge energy on a crude level, and he felt he was really coming along. Unfortunately, he also began to notice some side effects. These included: 1) Frightening hallucinations of his consciousness leaving his body and drifting uncontrollably away; 2) A feeling that things were moving much faster than they actually were (this was especially dangerous when he was driving); 3) Feeling his body become increasingly stiff internally; 4) Developing a thirst for power; 5) Feeling constantly hyper and unable to calm down; 6) Experiencing involuntary body spasms.

These problems were also beginning to occur to a friend of his, who happened to come to one of my classes. I noticed that he was essentially shredding himself and taught him to drain and repattern this vibrational energy. He in turn told Mike to come and see me.

By this time Mike had not been practicing for three years, yet most of his symptoms had not abated. He literally feared for his mental and physical health. I found that he had condensed the chi in his body, and through various techniques, including dissolving, I repatterned his energy and taught him how to continue this process at home. I also taught him techniques for removing the damaging chi from his body, techniques very similar to those found in this book. Two years later, his problems had pretty much resolved.

Discharging Energy

Many other qigong practices, such as discharging energy at a distance, are not inherently dangerous but do require a firm foundation in the grounding techniques described in this book. Most problems in qigong are the result of energy getting stuck and energy not flowing through the system. Knowing how to ground energy out can be a lifesaver. I should also add that much of the time, the action-at-a-distance qigong requires a good deal of cooperation among the participants, and there is a certain amount of exaggeration going on whenever this subject is discussed or demonstrated. These are methods for training a person's sensitivity to chi. It is virtually impossible to make a person with a developed will move or jump against his or her will by only projecting chi at a distance without physical contact.

The Dangers of Forcing and Fast Results

Qigong practices that give you a very rapid sense of increased physical or psychic power sometimes do so by overstraining the central nervous system. Qigong systems that promote an even, steady, upward curve of chi development are safer and usually more reliable for long-term progress. Extreme, forceful practices have the most consistently dangerous side-effects. If you undertake forceful practices, you should be supervised by regular ongoing weekly contact with a teacher who can adjust chi development to turn a potentially dangerous practice into a safe one. Shaolin practices are extremely forceful, so an ethical, experienced and knowledgeable teacher is a necessity.

If your body, mind, emotions, or psychic perceptions are getting weird or painful simply stop practicing until you find out clearly what is going on. Whatever your strength or capacity, your qigong practices must be internally comfortable. Forcing yourself radically beyond your individual limitations is usually what causes damage to your nerves, glands, internal organs, and brain. Overdoing internal energy practices may be compared to overtraining that causes external body damage in athletes. First and foremost find an honest, competent teacher who has your best interests at heart.

Most Qigong Is Safe

Notwithstanding all the previous warnings, most qigong systems are actually quite safe. Do not be afraid to practice qigong simply because some techniques may be dangerous. All valuable technologies have some element of danger. The purpose of this appendix is simply to open people's eyes to the negative aspects of qigong, which are commonly glossed over in our infatuation with things strange and foreign. I wish to reiterate that the material presented in this book and others I have written is the safest and most effective I have found in decades of research, both in Asia and the West.

APPENDIX D:

Techniques to Alleviate Tension and Discomfort While Sitting in a Chair

Here are three chair-sitting techniques that will help alleviate physical tension and pain, so you can focus on what you are doing rather than squirming or being distracted by physical discomfort. These techniques can be adapted for people practicing sitting qigong and meditation as well as for office workers, especially those using computers. The exercises that follow are reprinted from Chapter 3 of *The Great Stillness*.

1. When sitting in a chair, keep both feet flat on the floor, with the outsides of your feet being no wider than your shoulders. If you can, rest the palms of your hands on your knee-caps, your fingertips ideally pointing straight ahead. Your elbows should be bent and loose, not stiff-armed; keep your elbow tips gently moving downward toward your thighs. If you raise your elbows your shoulders will rise, and your spine will then tire more rapidly. Move your elbows gently to the sides. This move will create space inside your body where your spine can be more easily held straight. In an alternative method, place your palms along the body's centerline, directly in front of your lower tantien. Your palms may be touching surface to surface with hands lightly clasped, or the back of one hand may rest on the palm of the other, palms facing up (which hand is on top may be alternated over time). If at all possible, do not touch the backrest of the chair with your spine. Your body should be at ease, and your spine in particular should remain relaxed and straight. Figure 6-7 (p. 105) and Figure 6-9 (p. 106) show the correct alignments.

2. You may find that all these unsupported back positions are too straining or painful for your back or neck. If so, sit back in the chair as you slide down the backrest *(Figure 16-1A)*, and press your upper buttock muscles backward and upward to lift against the back of the chair *(Figures 16-1A and B)*. This motion allows your buttock and back muscles to connect without gaps. The motion pushes your buttock muscles up against the back of the chair *(Figure 16-1C)*, thereby providing a stabilizing support for your lower back. In contrast, if your buttock muscles push downward into the seat of the chair, the muscles of your lower back can also be pulled down. A downward muscle movement increases the

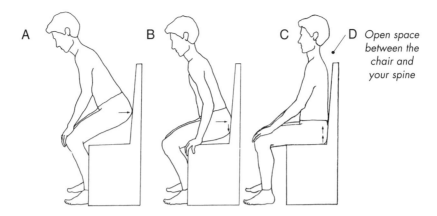

The Buttocks Support the Lower Back
Figure 16-1

arch of your lower back, compressing your vertebrae and straining your lower back muscles. This progression can then pull the vertebrae of your lower back out of alignment. So keep your spine straight, without any rounding or slumping. Keep your spine away from making contact with the middle and upper part of your chair's backrest *(Figure 16-1D)*. Only your rear end touches the back of the chair to push your lower back muscles upwards, adding back support.

3. If you still experience too much strain or physical pain, then allow your back to be fully supported by the back of the chair. This is best done in two stages. First, as you sit, consciously use the pressure of the chair against your back *(Figure 16-2A)* to keep as much space as possible between each of your vertebrae along the whole length of your spine.

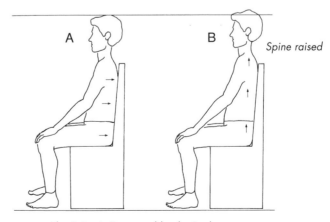

The Spine Is Supported by the Backrest
Figure 16-2

You can use the adhesive quality and friction of the fasciae of your back to stick to the chair's backrest, similar to the way a wet T-shirt sticks to your skin. (Fasciae are the connective tissues that bind your muscles together so they can function without being overly tight, slack or floppy.) Second, when being fully supported by a backrest, pay attention, at regular intervals, to equally lifting and lengthening all parts of the spine *(Figure 16-2B)*, with the idea of keeping the spinal cord lightly stretched and not compressed. Uneven compression of the spinal cord will eventually result in the back collapsing somewhere, straining muscles or causing vertebrae to misalign. Sitting correctly relieves these problems. Your sitting time should be spent working on your job or your internal meditation techniques, rather than squirming or being distracted by physical discomfort.

Sitting and Pain

The problem of pain brought about by prolonged sitting in a chair, whether in meditation or working at a desk, is caused by the progressive contraction and shortening of the deep muscles and fasciae from the bottom of the pelvis to the navel. If this contraction of the thighs, hips, and belly is strong enough, the strain will extend higher, and all the soft tissue between your head and your pelvis will be pulled downward. The longer you sit, the more the contracting originating in your pelvis will tighten and bring fatigue to the muscles, tendons, and vertebrae all the way up to your neck and shoulders, with the potential to cause any one of them to misalign. Contraction in your muscles, in turn, can overstretch your ligaments, stressing your hip and knee joints, causing pain.

The solution lies in stretching out the deep muscles and soft tissue (ligaments, tendons, and fasciae) from your knee to your kwa and lower belly at any time those tissues begin to shorten or fatigue *(see Figure 9-6, p. 163)*. You accomplish this stretching by making small movements of your pelvis and trunk during sitting. These movements reestablish the nerve signals to the offending muscles, instructing them to keep stretched and not collapse, thus preventing pain and fatigue. The trick is to maintain the spring of the soft tissues inside the kwa, by eliminating slack or involuntary contractions, and yet avoid becoming too taut.

Origin of Material in This Book

Opening the Energy Gates of Your Body is my own unique method of teaching traditional Taoist practices that I studied in depth over a more than a decade of training in China.

In 1968, I learned the outer form—the physical shell—of most material taught in this volume from my teacher Wang Shu Jin in Taiwan and his student Chang I Jung in Tokyo. I initially practiced this material five hours a day for five months, and then over the next eighteen years learned the internal components from various teachers and Taoist masters, including Hung I Hsiang and Huang Hsi I.

The standing posture is the most basic posture in qigong, and is found to some degree in all schools. It is the Taoist equivalent to the martial arts horse stance.

Cloud Hands is the basic exercise to connect the arms and legs to the spine. The First Swing, which energizes the lower organs, is found in almost all qigong systems. The Second Swing, which joins the legs to the spine and energizes the middle organs, is less common, and the Third Swing, which energizes the upper organs and the brain, is less common still. Historically, though, they should be done together. One swing alone may not be strong enough to cure a serious problem, but when done together and in the order presented, the effect is synergistic.

The Taoist Spine Stretch was the only movement I did not originally learn from Wang, but over the past 3,000 years, some schools have included it in this sequence. It is the beginning move of traditional spinal qigong. In its entirety, spinal qigong teaches how to bring energy up the spine, connect the spine to the rest of the body, completely control vertebral movement, and access the cerebrospinal pump, which purely deals with the spine.

Some of the internal components of these exercises have been included in this volume, with more details in other books in my Living Taoism collection. Some of the internal energetic work, it should be pointed out, can only safely be learned under the supervision of a master, and I have only described here what can be presented to the public without danger.

I had the help of many masters, some of whom I cannot mention by name because of the political situation in China. Others I cannot mention because it was their expressed wish to depart the world "without leaving any footprints." I could, however, never have understood the complete picture without having been formally adopted by Liu Hung Chieh and accepted as his disciple. Liu filled in the gaps in my education, as well as teaching me much less common material that came from his ten years of training with Taoist adepts in the mountains of Western China, rather than from his martial arts background.

Liu Hung Chieh's Education as a Taoist Master

Liu Hung Chieh began to study martial arts at the age of 12. After three years of training in Shaolin style kung fu, he was accepted as the youngest formal disciple by the Beijing Bagua School. At this time, he also learned hsing-i from members of the school and outside teachers. In 1928, he represented the Beijing Bagua School at the first All-China Martial Arts Competition, which had to be stopped due to excessive injuries.

In the mid-1930s, Liu, was head of instructors at the Hunan Branch of the Central Government's National Martial Arts Association. Two of his junior instructors at the time were Wu Jien Chuan's sons, and from them he learned Wu style tai chi. Later, Liu became Wu Jien Chuan's formal disciple, and lived in Wu's house in Hong Kong. Because of Liu's strong internal martial arts background, Wu was able to teach him the deepest levels of the Wu style.

When Liu returned to the Chinese mainland he studied with the abbot Tan Hsu Fa Shi, and was declared formally enlightened according to the tenets of Tien Tai Buddhism. He then spent ten years studying with Taoist masters in Szechuan Province in Western China, completing the practice for becoming one with the Tao.

With the ascension of Communism in China, he returned to Beijing, where he lived out the rest of his life quietly, teaching only a few students, and perfecting his practices.

APPENDIX F:

About the Romanization of Chinese Words in This Book

Any attempt to transliterate the sounds of Chinese words into English with any accuracy will fall far short. This is because Chinese not only has sounds that English does not have, but also uses a system of vocal "tones," which do not exist in English. Furthermore, English has sounds that are not present in Chinese. English speakers attempting to pronounce Chinese words will invariably add sounds from their own language, which will distort the pronunciation of Chinese.

None of the major systems for Romanizing Chinese words is very accurate. Written Chinese is composed of ideogram pictures, each of which may convey one idea or several combined ideas. These ideograms, when spoken, are pronounced differently in the different Chinese languages. To the foreign ear, these languages can sometimes seem as different as French and German. For example, the word for family is jia in the "National Language" (Mandarin, or common-people speech), but it is gar in Cantonese, a regional Chinese sublanguage, or dialect, spoken by over sixty million people in the province of Canton (Guangzhou) and by the people of Hong Kong. There are yet more regional languages, again with different sounds for the same character, such as Szechuanese (which more people speak than Cantonese) and Minnanhua of Fukien province (which is an older language than Cantonese). To make matters worse, there are subdialects within each major dialect. In some instances in Old China, people from the same province only one or two hundred miles away from each other could hardly communicate with each other.

This linguistic mess stymied communication throughout China for thousands of years, with the written language (in a mostly illiterate nation) being the only common means of communication. As all power in Old China came from the Emperor and his bureaucracy, over time the language of Beijing became the common medium of communication through-out China for the educated. After the Emperors fell, both the Nationalist government and, later, the Communist government made the language of Beijing—still the seat of government—the national language of China and called it the Common People's speech, which, in English, is called Mandarin Chinese (from the days of the Emperors). Mandarin, as the official language of all of China, is now what truly can be called Chinese, which every single person in China learns to speak. Throughout this book, all Chinese terms used are in Mandarin and not in the regional dialects.

The Westerner who has no idea how to speak Chinese (and probably little interest in learning) is now bombarded with multiple systems of transliteration for the exact same sound, including the Pinyin system, the Wade-Giles system and the Yale system. In both the Wade-Giles system (invented by German monks, used in the old days by translators who mostly could only read Chinese but not speak it, and now used by the Nationalists in Taiwan), and the Pinyin system (developed for use inside China by the Chinese when the Communist government was trying to raise the literacy rate in China), many of the written English transliterations when pronounced do not sound anything like the Chinese sounds. The only Romanization system that was created to mimic as closely as possible the Chinese language using the English phonetic system was the Yale system, created at Yale University specifically to teach English speakers how to speak Chinese.

For example, qigong in the Yale system is chi gung; in Pinyin, it is qigong or qi gong; and in the Wade-Giles, it is chi kung. Actually, the way it is said in China is closest to chee gung. The qi of the Pinyin and the kung of the Wade-Giles are not accurate in terms of how this spelling would normally be pronounced in English.

This language lesson may seem academic to some. However, there are over a billion Chinese in the world and miscommunication can waste a lot of time and energy. This book uses transliterations that are either the ones most commonly used or that allow the English speaker to best mimic what the Chinese actually sounds like. Thus, I have not been concerned with adhering strictly to any one formal transliteration system.

APPENDIX G:

Taoism: A Living Tradition

Many traditions that are based on ancient philosophies and religions have vibrantly continued into modern times. Because they manifest in our lives today, they are called living traditions. These include Christianity, Islam, Judaism, Buddhism, Vedanta and Taoism. The latter three actively practice physical exercises and energy work.

Taoism is the least known of the living traditions. Although its main literary works—the *I Ching*, the writings of Chuang Tse and the *Tao Te Ching* by Lao Tse—are well known and available in many translations, the practical methods and techniques of implementing Taoist philosophy in daily life are little documented in the West.

One branch of living Taoist philosophy is about developing and using one's personal chi or life force energy to strengthen, heal and benefit oneself and others. This branch encompasses two broad traditions: the Water and the Fire. The Water tradition, based on the philosophies of Lao Tse, emphasizes effort without force, relaxation and letting go, as a flow of water slowly erodes rock. The Fire tradition, developed 1,500 years later, emphasizes force, pushing forward and breaking through barriers.

The Taoist lineages that Bruce Frantzis holds are in the Water tradition, which has received little exposure in the West. Part of his lineage empowers and directs him to bring practices based on that tradition to Westerners. He learned the Chinese language and became immersed in the traditions of China during his training there.

While Frantzis studied with his main teacher, Grandmaster Liu Hung Chieh, texts were presented as: "This is what they say; this is what they mean; this is how to do them." Frantzis offers an unprecedented bridge to this pragmatic approach to spirituality; in fact, we are not aware of any other English or European language source for this style of teaching. It means that spirituality is not just an aspiration for which people strive in the dark—"in a mirror, darkly"—to quote St. Paul, but it can become a genuine, accomplishable reality.

The Frantzis Energy Arts System

Drawing on 16 years of training in Asia, Bruce Frantzis has developed a practical, comprehensive system of programs that can enable people of all ages and fitness levels to increase their core energy and attain vibrant health.

Core Qigong Practices

The Frantzis Energy Arts System® includes six primary qigong courses that, together with the Longevity Breathing program, progressively and safely incorporate all the aspects of neigong—the original chi cultivation (qigong) system in China that originated from the Taoists. Although the qigong techniques are very old, Bruce Frantzis' system of teaching them is unique. It is specifically tailored to Westerners and the needs of modern life. A good analogy is that Frantzis has created the cup—the Frantzis Energy Arts system—that can hold the wine—these ancient Taoist practices.

The core practices consist of:

Longevity Breathing
Dragon and Tiger Qigong
Opening the Energy Gates of Your Body Qigong
The Marriage of Heaven and Earth Qigong
Bend the Bow Spinal Qigong
Spiraling Energy Body Qigong
Gods Playing in the Clouds Qigong

The core qigong programs were deliberately chosen because they are among the oldest, most effective and most treasured of Taoist energy practices. They are ideal for progressively incorporating the major components of neigong in a manner that is comprehensible and understandable to Westerners. They provide students with the foundation necessary for clearly and systematically learning and advancing their practice in Taoist energy arts.

Longevity Breathing Program

Frantzis has developed this method to teach authentic Taoist breathing in systematic stages. Breathing with the whole body has been used for millennia to enhance the ability to dissolve and release energy blockages in the mind/body, enhancing well-being and spiritual awareness. Incorporating these breathing techniques into any other Taoist energy practice will help bring out its full potential.

Dragon and Tiger Medical Qigong

This is one of the most direct and accessible low-impact qigong healing methods that China has produced. This 1500-year-old form of medical qigong affects the human body in a manner similar to acupuncture. Its seven simple movements can be done by virtually anyone, whatever their state of health.

Opening the Energy Gates of Your Body Qigong

This program introduces 3,000-year-old qigong techniques that are fundamental to advancing any energy arts practice. Core exercises teach you the basic body alignments and how to increase your internal awareness of chi in your body and dissolve blocked energy.

Marriage of Heaven and Earth Qigong

This qigong incorporates techniques widely used in China to help heal back, neck, spine and joint problems. It is especially effective for helping to mitigate repetitive stress injury and carpal tunnel problems. This program teaches some important neigong components, including openings and closings (pulsing), more complex breathing techniques and how to move chi through the energy channels of the body.

Bend the Bow Spinal Qigong

Bend the Bow Spinal Qigong continues the work of strengthening and regenerating the spine that is learned in Marriage of Heaven and Earth Qigong. This program incorporates neigong components for awakening and controlling the energies of the spine.

Spiraling Energy Body Qigong

This advanced program teaches you to dramatically raise your energy level and master how energy moves in circles and spirals throughout your body. It incorporates neigong components for: directing the upward flow of energy; projecting chi along the body's spiraling pathways; delivering or projecting energy at will to or from any part of the body; and activating the body's left, right and central channels and the micro-cosmic orbit.

Gods Playing in the Clouds Qigong

Gods Playing in the Clouds incorporates some of the oldest and most powerful Taoist rejuvenation techniques. This program amplifies all the physical, breathing and energetic components learned in earlier qigong programs and completes the process of integrating all the components of neigong. It is also the final stage of learning to strengthen and balance the energies of your three tantiens, central energy channel and spine. Gods Playing in the Clouds Qigong serves as a spiritual bridge to Taoist meditation.

Tai Chi and Bagua as Health Arts

Tai chi and bagua practiced as health arts intensify the benefits of the core qigong practices.

Most Westerners learn tai chi purely as a health exercise rather than a martial art. Like all qigong programs, tai chi relaxes and regulates the central nervous system, releasing physical and emotional stress, and promoting mental and emotional well-being. Tai chi's gentle, non-jarring movements are ideal for people of any age and body type and can give them a high degree of relaxation, balance and physical coordination.

Even more ancient than tai chi, the circle walking techniques of bagua were developed over four thousand years ago in Taoist monasteries as a health and meditation art. The techniques open up the possibilities of the mind to achieve stillness and clarity; generate a strong, healthy, disease-free body; and, perhaps more importantly, maintain internal balance while either your inner world or the events of the external world are rapidly changing.

Longevity Breathing Yoga

Taoist yoga is ancient China's soft yet powerful alternative to what is popularly known today as Hatha yoga. The system Frantzis has developed to teach this is called Longevity Breathing® Yoga. Its primary emphasis is to stimulate the flow of chi and free up any blocked energy. Combining gentle postures and Longevity Breathing techniques systematically opens the body's energy channels, thereby activating and stimulating chi flow. Postures are held from two to five minutes and require virtually no muscular effort, enabling you to easily focus on what is internal so you can feel where the chi is blocked and gently free it up.

Healing Others with Qigong Tui Na

Part of Frantzis' Taoist training was to become a Chinese doctor, primarily using the qigong healing techniques known as qigong tui na. During this training period, he worked with more than 10,000 patients. Frantzis no longer works as a qigong doctor, either privately or in clinics, but occasionally offers training in therapeutic healing techniques.

Qigong tui na is a special branch of Chinese medicine that is designed to unblock, free and balance chi in others. You learn to project energy from your hands, voice and eyes to facilitate healing using 200 hand techniques. You also learn how to avoid burnout from your therapeutic practice. To heal others, you must first learn to unblock and free your own chi and to control the specific pathways through which it flows.

Shengong

Whereas *chi* or *qi* means "energy," shen means "spirit." Spirit equals meditation, which equals spirituality. So the term shengong literally means "spirit work."

Chi practices can make your body healthier and physically stronger. Meditation is about going beyond the energy of your flesh and internal organs where the primal or instinctual emotions reside. In terms of meditation, shengong is the fusion of qigong with the emotional, mental, psychic, karmic energy bodies to the level of your essence. This is the point at which you move into Taoist meditation.

Tao Meditation

Frantzis is a lineage holder in the gentle Water method of Taoist meditation passed down from the teachings of Lao Tse over 2,500 years ago. Bruce calls the technique he has developed to teach this tradition Tao meditation. Taoist meditation is little known in the West and is often confused with Buddhism. In Taoism, the road to spirituality involves more than having health, calmness and a stable, peaceful mind. These are just the necessary prerequisites and are achieved through qigong, Longevity Breathing, tai chi and other Taoist energy programs.

Tao Meditation includes using chi to help you release anxieties, expectations, and negative emotions—referred to as blockages—that prevent you from feeling truly alive and joyful. The first goal is to address spiritual responsibility for yourself, helping you become a relaxed, spontaneous, fully mature and open human being. A second goal is awakening the great human potential inside you, fostering compassion and balance. The third is reaching inner stillness—a place deep inside you that is absolutely permanent and stable. As your practice deepens, the 16-part neigong system is brought into play to accelerate the evolutionary spiritual process.

Tai Chi as Meditation

Tai chi is commonly referred to as moving meditation. Tai chi's slow, graceful movements provide relaxed focus, quiet down your internal dialogue and engender a deep sense of relaxation that helps release inner tensions.

Only a few tai chi masters know how to transform the practice of tai chi to a complete

Taoist moving meditation. Liu Hung Chieh taught Frantzis this tradition and empowered him to teach it.

Internal Martial Arts

The internal martial arts teach you to use relaxation, chi, and stillness of mind to accomplish the pragmatic goal of winning in a violent confrontation, rather than using muscular tension or anger for power.

Tai Chi Chuan

Tai chi is a potent martial art. Frantzis trained extensively in the traditional Wu, Yang and Chen styles of tai chi chuan, including short and long forms, push hands, self-defense techniques and such traditional weapons as sticks and swords.

Bagua Zhang

Bagua was designed to fight up to eight opponents at once. Virtually no other martial art system or style, internal or external, has combined and seamlessly integrated into one package the whole pantheon of martial arts fighting techniques as effectively as bagua.

Bagua is first and foremost an art of internal energy movement that embodies the eight primal energies that are encompassed by the eight trigrams of the *I Ching*. The basic internal power training consists of learning eight palm changes and combining them with walking, spiraling and twisting arm movements and constant changes of direction.

Hsing-I Chuan

Hsing-i (also transliterated as xing yi) emphasizes all aspects of the mind to create its forms and fighting movements. It is an equally potent healing practice because it makes people healthy and then very strong.

Its five basic movements are related to the five primal elements or phases of energy—metal, water, wood, fire and earth—upon which Chinese medicine is based and from which all manifested phenomena are created. Hsing-i's training is based on a linear, militaristic approach: marching in straight lines, with a powerful emphasis at the end of every technique on mentally or physically taking an enemy down.

Living Taoism Collection

The purpose of Bruce Frantzis' Living Taoism™ Collection is not to repeat or interpret ancient texts, but rather to show how Taoist practices are alive and extremely relevant to modern life. As personal health and energy systems, they can benefit you profoundly.

Books

Other books in the Living Taoism Collection include *Tai Chi: Health for Life*; *The Power of Internal Martial Arts and Chi*; *Bagua and Tai Chi: Exploring the Potential of Chi, Martial Arts, Meditation and the I-Ching;* and two volumes on the water method of Taoist meditation, *Relaxing into Your Being* and *The Great Stillness*. Frantzis' latest meditation book is *Tao of Letting Go: Meditation for Modern Living,* a companion to the CD-set described in the next section. *Chi Revolution* describes how chi is the power behind spirituality, meditation, sexual vitality, acupuncture, internal martial arts and the divination methods of the *I Ching*. It includes the Chi Rev Workout™, a simple but potent exercise program, much of which is derived from Dragon and Tiger Qigong. *Dragon and Tiger Medical Qigong: Develop Health and Energy in 7 Simple Movements* contains detailed instructions of this set's movements, energy mechanics and breathing techniques, with more than 650 illustrations (laminated poster available).

CDs and DVDs

DVD titles range from a general introduction to Taoist practices, *Taoist Energy Arts,* to specific instructional programs such as Longevity Breathing.

The Tao of Letting Go, a six-CD set, is a complete meditation course. For the first time in the West, Frantzis shares the Inner Dissolving method of Tao meditation. This special recording introduces you to how powerfully meditation can help you let go of tension, fear, anger and pain. Frantzis guides you through turning inwards to awaken the great human potential inside yourself and move closer to feeling truly alive and joyful.

Frantzis has recently released a three-CD set, *Ancient Songs of the Tao,* a collection of never-before-recorded chants in ancient Chinese. These Taoist liturgies are used to balance and transform the energetic frequencies within a human being. You can listen to them while performing any movement or meditation practice. The songs can help you breathe fully into your entire body and optimize your heath and well-being.

In *Strings of the Tao* Frantzis chants powerful liturgies accompanied by Kitaro violinist, Steve Kindler. Taoist exercises for better sex, vibrant health and longevity are described in the 2-CD set, *Chi Gung (Qigong) for the Sexes.*

Training Opportunities

Bruce Frantzis is the founder of Energy Arts, Inc., based in Marin County, California. Energy Arts offers instructor certification programs, retreats, corporate and public workshops, and lectures worldwide. Frantzis teaches Energy Arts courses in qigong, Longevity Breathing, the internal martial arts of tai chi, bagua and hsing-i; Longevity Breathing Yoga; the healing techniques of qigong tui na; and the Water method of Taoist meditation.

Comprehensive online training courses are also available. Topics may include meditation, bagua, tai chi and qigong. See EnergyArts.com for current programs.

Instructor Certification

Prior training in Frantzis Energy Arts programs is a requirement for most instructor courses. The certification process is rigorous to ensure that instructors teach the authentic traditions inherent in these arts.

Train with a Frantzis Energy Arts Certified Instructor

The Energy Arts Web site, EnergyArts.com, contains a directory of all the certified instructors worldwide. Since Bruce Frantzis no longer offers regular ongoing classes, he recommends locating an instructor in your area for regular training and for building on or preparing for his teachings.

Contact Information

Energy Arts, Inc.
P. O. Box 99
Fairfax, CA 94978-0099 USA
Phone: (415) 454-5243
Fax: (415) 454-0907

Visit EnergyArts.com to:

- Join our list to get free articles and audio material by Bruce Frantzis.
- Receive the latest details on events and training materials.
- See video clips of qigong and martial arts forms.
- Find a certified instructor near you or learn how to become one.
- Inquire about hosting a workshop or speaking engagement.

Read Bruce's personal blog at **TaiChiMaster.com**

Index